Counselling
in
Obstetrics and Gynaecology

Myra Hunter

Communication and Counselling in Health Care
Series editor: Hilton Davis

Counselling
in
Obstetrics and Gynaecology

Myra Hunter

Senior Research Fellow, Guy's Hospital Medical School
Head of Psychological Services to Obstetrics and Gynaecology,
University College Hospitals, London

Medical advisor: Wendy Savage
Senior Lecturer, The Royal London Hospital

 Published by the British Psychological Society

First published in 1994 by BPS Books (The British Psychological Society),
St Andrews House, 48 Princess Road East, Leicester LE1 7DR.

Distributed exclusively in North America by Paul H. Brookes Publishing Co., Inc.,
P.O. Box 10624, Baltimore, Maryland 21285, U.S.A.

A catalogue record for this book is available from the British Library.

ISBN 1 85433 119 1 paperback

Phototypeset by Gem Graphics, Trenance, Mawgan Porth, Cornwall

OTHER TITLES IN THE SERIES
Counselling Parents of Children with Chronic Illness or Disability
by Hilton Davis
Counselling for Heart Disease by Paul Bennett

Communication and Counselling in Health Care
Series editor: Hilton Davis

Counselling
in
Obstetrics and Gynaecology

Myra Hunter

Senior Research Fellow, Guy's Hospital Medical School
Head of Psychological Services to Obstetrics and Gynaecology,
University College Hospitals, London

Medical advisor: Wendy Savage
Senior Lecturer, The Royal London Hospital

BPS
BOOKS Published by the British Psychological Society

First published in 1994 by BPS Books (The British Psychological Society),
St Andrews House, 48 Princess Road East, Leicester LE1 7DR.

Distributed exclusively in North America by Paul H. Brookes Publishing Co., Inc.,
P.O. Box 10624, Baltimore, Maryland 21285, U.S.A.

A catalogue record for this book is available from the British Library.

ISBN 1 85433 119 1 paperback

Phototypeset by Gem Graphics, Trenance, Mawgan Porth, Cornwall

OTHER TITLES IN THE SERIES
Counselling Parents of Children with Chronic Illness or Disability
by Hilton Davis
Counselling for Heart Disease by Paul Bennett

CONTENTS

Preface to the series   VIII
Foreword by Wendy Savage   IX

Introduction   1

1. THEORIES AND PRACTICES   4
Cultural influences   4
Historical influences   6
Twentieth century developments   7
A biopsychosocial model   9
Summary   15

2. EXPERIENCES OF REPRODUCTIVE PROBLEMS   16
The perception of symptoms   16
The consultation   18
Investigations and minor operations   21
   Abortion or termination of pregnancy   22
   Cervical screening   23
Major surgery   25
The experience of childbirth   28
Infertility: investigations and treatment   31
Problems of the reproductive cycle   34
Chronic reproductive problems   40
   Pelvic pain   40
   Gynaecological cancer   42
Bereavement and pregnancy loss   43
Summary   48

3. COUNSELLING: DEFINITIONS, AIMS, PROCESS   49
Aims of counselling   50
The relationship: expert or helper   50
The counselling process   52
Summary   59

4. INITIAL CONTACT AND EXPLORATION   60
The setting   60
Attending and listening   62
Demonstrating empathy   66
Problem clarification   69
Further exploration   72
Case studies   74
Dealing with distress   80
Dealing with anger   82

The need to practice   85
Summary   86

5. PROVIDING INFORMATION AND SUPPORT   87
Guidelines for providing information   87
Giving bad news   89
Preparation for investigations   92
Preparation for surgery   95
Support before, during and after childbirth   97
Pregnancy loss   99
Summary   104

6. NEW PERSPECTIVES AND PROBLEM-SOLVING   105
New perspectives and alternative models   105
Problem-solving   109
Assertiveness and stress management   112
Case studies   113
Maintaining changes   122
When and how to end counselling?   123
Dealing with the health care system   125
Health promotion   126
Summary   128

7. CONCLUSIONS   129
Principles of communication and counselling   129
Evaluation of counselling   129
Support for health workers   132
Summary   136

Appendix A: Organizations and support groups   137
Appendix B: Relaxation and breathing exercises   140
References   141
Index   146

LIST OF FIGURES AND TABLES

Figure 1.1: A biopsychosocial model of reproductive problems   9
Table 5.1: How to break bad news   90
Table 5.2: Helping people to make informed choices   94
Table 6.1: Managing stress   113

This book is dedicated to my daughters, Clara and Meirian.

ACKNOWLEDGEMENTS

I would like to thank all the women, and couples, who I have met in different health-care settings, and from whom I have learnt so much. I am particularly grateful to Laura and Heather Tomlinson, Joan Hogg, Sheila Lawler, Jane Harris, Edana Mingella, Caroline Barry, Noel Walker, Linda Long, Lesley Bulman, Julia Feast and Liz Hopper for sharing their thoughts and experiences. Many thanks also to Rochelle Serwator at BPS Books, John Weinman, Professor of Psychology at Guy's Medical School, and to Hilton Davis for his constructive and helpful comments.

Preface to the Series

People who suffer chronic disease or disability are confronted by problems that are as much psychological as physical, and involve all members of their family and the wider social network. Psychosocial adaptation is important in its own right, in terms of making necessary changes in life style, altering aspirations or coping with an uncertain future. However, it may also influence the effectiveness of the diagnostic and treatment processes, and hence eventual outcomes.

As a consequence, health care, whether preventive or treatment-oriented, must encompass the psychosocial aspects of illness as well as the physical, at all phases of the life cycle and at all stages of disease. The basis of this is skilled communication and supportive counselling by all involved in providing services, professionally or voluntarily. Everyone, from the student to the experienced practitioner, can benefit from appropriate training in this area, where the social skills required are complex and uncertain.

Although there is a sizeable research literature related to counselling and communication in the area of health care, specialist texts for training purposes are scarce. The current series was, therefore, conceived as a practical resource for all who work in health services. Each book is concerned with a specific area of health care. The authors have been asked to provide detailed information, from the patient's perspective, about the problems (physical, psychological and social) faced by patients and their families. Each book examines the role of counselling and communication in the process of helping people to come to terms and deal with these problems, and presents usable frameworks as a guide to the helping process. Detailed and practical descriptions of the major qualities, abilities and skills that are required to provide the most effective help for patients are included.

The intention is to stimulate professional and voluntary helpers alike to explore their efforts at supportive communication. It is hoped that by so doing, they become sufficiently aware of patient difficulties and the processes of adaptation, and more able to facilitate positive adjustment. The aims of the series will have been met if patients and their families feel someone has listened and if they feel respected in their struggle for health. A central theme is the effort to make people feel better about themselves and able to face the future, no matter how bleak, with dignity.

Hilton Davis
Series editor

Foreword

It has been a pleasure to read this book, which should be of great help to health professionals. Dealing with women who have problems associated with fertility, birth and the parts of the body relating to reproduction and sexuality, is an emotional process, yet all too often these matters are dealt with in a mechanistic way.

It is only 25 years since Bourne's study of general practitioners' attitudes towards women who had delivered a stillborn baby, showed how stillbirths tend to be 'forgotten'. Since then the midwifery and obstetric professions, with the help of Bourne and Lewis and self-help groups such as SANDS, have learnt that parents need to be able to see and hold their dead baby, to be able to name and bury the child, and grieve in just the same way as for an older person who dies. SANDS is the offspring of the organization founded by Hazelanne Lewis, a social worker who had herself experienced the loss of a baby and the inability of the medical profession to deal with this in those days.

Pitt, who in the same year as Bourne, 1968, published a classic study of depression in pregnancy, is one of a band of psychiatrists and psychologists who have worked with obstetricians and gynaecologists, to help us understand the importance of psychology in our field. Kumar continued this work in the 1980s, looking at the interaction of antenatal and postnatal depression. He is a founder member of the Marce Society, an organization which has brought together workers in all fields interested in the study of puerperal mental illness, and helped to co-ordinate the research in this area.

This book is based on the practical experience of the author, and recent research on the psychosocial needs of women receiving maternity and gynaecological care. The word 'counselling' is used in many different ways. This book emphasizes the use of a non-directive communication style, information giving and emotional support in a problem-solving framework. Such counselling is crucial to the effectiveness of care and women's satisfaction with their consultations. This approach can be hard for doctors to accept, as they are used to making decisions on behalf of sick people. However, in recent years it has gained ground, and this text will be very valuable for those training as future specialists, general practitioners, nurses and midwives.

This book ought to be widely used and, I hope, it will facilitate the growing understanding of the importance of psychological and emotional factors in obstetrics and gynaecology, and so help health professionals to provide better care for women.

Wendy Savage   July 1993

Introduction

When asked about obstetrics and gynaecology, almost every woman has her tale to tell; embarrassment, misunderstandings and discomfort are common reactions to menstrual, reproductive and gynaecological experiences.

'After I had the baby I was exhausted and tearful. Tom (the baby) had one complication after another, I just wanted to cry. It was just not what I'd expected.'

'The worst part of it (being in a gynaecological ward for infertility investigations) was being treated like a non-person. The staff were very kind but didn't really look me in the eye or ask me what I felt about it all.'

'I've had flooding (heavy menstrual bleeding) for the last year. It's getting worse and for half the month I worry about when it's going to start. When the flooding starts I have to be very careful and often try to organize things so that I stay at home.'

Normal developmental changes such as menstruation, pregnancy and the menopause often require emotional and practical adjustments, but when systems do not function as expected, as in the case of infertility, pelvic pain or menorrhagia, a woman's sense of well-being and her quality of life may well be adversely affected. However, the emphasis here is not upon the individual woman as victim of her reproductive changes. Many consultations in obstetrics and gynaecology are not about illness at all, but concern the exchange of information and the need for decision-making, such as in antenatal and family planning clinics. It is often in the communication with health care professionals about reproductive and gynaecological changes that many women experience lack of understanding and insensitivity.

Broad definitions of both problems and counselling will be adopted. Counselling will include communication skills, as well as problem-focused counselling. Problems will refer to difficulties encountered during consultations and possibly arising as a result of treatments, in addition to symptoms that women might bring to health care workers.

The aim is not to view normal developmental processes as medical problems, but to highlight areas of difficulty in understanding and communication in the hope of alleviating unnecessary distress. The broad term 'reproductive problems' will be used here and in the following chapters to refer to specific obstetric and gynaecological symptoms and chronic disorders, as well as problems arising from medical interventions.

The main message of this book is to help those involved in women's health care to understand the nature of reproductive problems and to communicate effectively so that appropriate solutions can be reached. Three principles will be emphasized:

• Women and health care workers attempt to communicate as equals.
• In order to make informed decisions, women should be told clearly about their problem and its treatment.
• Women should be given as much control of their treatment as possible.

There are at least three main reasons why counselling skills are essential in this area of health care.

1. Talking with women about their personal lives and intimate parts of their bodies requires much sensitivity and skill, and the ability to listen. It is in this first stage of consultation that women often feel uncomfortable and misunderstood.

2. Studies have found that women attending gynaecological clinics report high levels of emotional distress (Byrne, 1984; Worsley *et al.*, 1977); higher than those in the general population or in women attending other out-patient clinics. A variety of explanations have been offered for this, and more than one explanation is probably needed.

For some, distress will result from the gynaecological symptoms themselves. It is also possible that women who are already distressed may be more likely to develop symptoms, or be more sensitive to reproductive problems or changes. Experience of sexual abuse can, in some cases, lead to both physical and emotional problems.

It is well known that depression is twice as prevalent in women when compared with men, and this is particularly true for women during the child-bearing years (Weissman and Klerman, 1981; Briscoe, 1982). Both psychosocial and biological theories have been put forward to explain this difference. However, there seems to be much more evidence to support psychosocial explanations of depression in women than for explanations based on hormonal causes.

Decisions to seek medical help are thus influenced by many

complex psychological and social factors, often unrelated to specific disease processes. Counselling skills are essential if health care workers and others are to understand the reasons for seeking help, the psychosocial context in which problems arise, and the impact of gynaecological problems upon a woman's sense of well-being.

3. The development of family planning clinics, well woman clinics, breast and cervical screening services and routine obstetric care has meant that large numbers of women across a range of ages come into contact with health care workers. The opportunity exists in these settings for the provision of health education and for preventative interventions, but this can only be achieved with good communication.

In the next chapter, past and current theories about 'women's problems' are discussed in relation to stages of the reproductive cycle: menstruation, pregnancy, childbirth and the menopause. A bio-psychosocial model is presented which includes the main factors that influence physical and emotional well-being, as well as help-seeking behaviour.

In Chapter 2 a wide range of reproductive problems is described. While facts and figures are provided, the major concern is to convey an understanding of the feelings, concerns and reactions of women in these circumstances.

The focus, in the rest of the book, is on the basic skills of communication and counselling. Practical guidelines are provided to help health care workers – be they midwives, nurses, doctors, social workers, health visitors or voluntary workers – to improve their communication skills, to be able to offer counselling and support when needed, as well as to face and deal more confidently with difficult situations. The value of good communication has always been accepted in medicine and is now being recognized as having a positive effect on recovery from illness, in reducing and preventing unnecessary distress, and in improving patient satisfaction. This book aims to bring together the principles and skills of counselling to address the particular problems encountered both by women and health care workers in obstetrics and gynaecology.

1

Theories and Practices

Theories, medical treatments and popular traditions surrounding reproduction and menstruation have varied appreciably over time and differ across cultures. Examples from the past and from different cultures described in this chapter give a broader perspective on current views and practices. A dominant theme, in the past and present, is for reproduction to be seen as a cause of psychological problems. Theories also tend to be one-dimensional, emphasizing either biological or social factors, and, as a result, understanding and treatment of women's problems has been inadequate and often unhelpful.

A multidimensional or biopsychosocial model is described at the end of this chapter. This model brings together the various cultural, social, psychological and biological factors that influence women's experiences of reproductive changes and problems. An approach to understanding the individual person who is seeking help, based on this model, will be used in the chapters that follow.

Cultural Influences

The menstrual taboo has existed in most parts of the world at some time and reflects an almost universally negative attitude towards menstrual blood. For example, specific beliefs imbue menstruating women with evil and destructive powers; they have been seen to cause male impotence, damage to crops and as a source of bad luck. As a result, in some cultures, women have been excluded from activities and sometimes isolated during and after menstruation. However, in many cultures, even where menstruation is taboo, menarche is the occasion for special ceremony signifying the onset of fertility and sexuality. While the taboo may well have a negative impact upon a young woman's ideas about female identity, she at least gains an external validation of her bodily changes.

In most western societies, although no overt rituals take place, menarche similarly brings the mixed message that a girl has become a woman, but that her menstrual blood and, by extension, her genitals are somewhat unpleasant and dirty. Young women today are still often embarrassed about buying sanitary towels or tampons, and advertisements which repeatedly stress the need for cleanliness and concealment reinforce such ideas. Ambivalent attitudes towards female sexuality are subtly learnt. For example, female genitals are often not acknowledged or even named, and their functions may not be understood or may be confused with excretion. Uncertainty about their developing bodies and conflict about sexual feelings are not uncommon amongst young women. One the one hand they are expected to be clean and pure, while there is also much social pressure to be physically attractive to men.

So, in many cultures a woman's early experiences of reproductive changes evoke embarrassment, humiliation and sometimes pain. The negative meanings of menstruation are also likely to have harmful effects on her self-image (see Ussher, 1989).

In certain cultures, the time after the menopause tends to be welcomed, as it can bring relief from repeated pregnancies, and sometimes greater social freedom. Cross-cultural studies have found that in cultures where the menopause is not seen as a medical problem, for example in South East Asia, women report fewer problems. Surprisingly, no word for hot flushes exists in the language of Mayan Indian women, who generally feel positive about the menopause (Beyenne, 1986). Dietary and lifestyle factors might also play a part in explanations of these striking cultural differences.

In western societies, where youth and beauty are highly valued, reaching the menopause is generally seen as a sign of ageing and decline, and the menopause has even been described as an oestrogen deficiency disease. Women in western cultures tend to report more symptoms, such as hot flushes and night sweats, and attribute more physical and emotional problems to this reproductive stage.

Cultural and economic factors also determine attitudes towards fertility and childbirth as well as expectations of family size. For example, in colonial America, when population growth was encouraged, it was not uncommon for women to have up to 12 children. As a result, those who were unmarried or infertile in their mid-twenties were treated as economically useless. The extent of medical intervention varies across cultures, as does the position women adopt to give birth. In one survey, 82 per cent of women in a sample of 76 cultures gave birth standing up or sitting or squatting, with only 18 per cent having their babies lying down (Oakley, 1979).

Childbirth is now seen as a medical rather than a social event in the western world, but again there are variations in medical practice between countries. For example, home births are much more common in Holland than in Germany, Sweden, Canada or Japan. Surgical interventions tend to be more prevalent in North American deliveries. In the 1980s, episiotomy (a cut made in the perineum during childbirth) was common practice and in 1990 the Caesarian section was the most commonly performed operation in the United States, closely followed by hysterectomy (Payer, 1989). One baby in four in the US and one in five in Canada are delivered by Caesarian section compared with seven per cent in the Netherlands.

Historical Influences

The menstrual taboo has existed for centuries, at least as far back as the birth of the major religions. From Graeco-Roman times until the 19th century, menstrual blood was widely thought to be retained in the body, destroying the body from within and causing an array of emotional and physical problems. There were remedies or treatments aimed at ensuring menstrual flow; heavy bleeding was valued! Purgatives, enemas and leeches were used in an attempt to delay the menopause.

Longstanding myths link the womb with emotionality. Psychological and health problems in women have even been attributed to the belief that the womb moved around the body causing inner turmoil!

It was in the 19th century, however, that the reproductive cycle became more clearly associated with disease. Victorian psychiatrists developed theories about female insanity that were specifically linked to the female life cycle. Puberty, menstruation, childbirth and menopause were regarded as crucial times during which the mind is weakened. The diagnosis of involutional melancholia, which has since been deemed invalid, was used to describe psychosis thought to be caused by the menopause. The psychosocial context, such as the constraints and restricted lifestyles experienced by women in Victorian times tended to be overlooked.

In Europe, during the latter half of the 19th century, many emotional as well as physical symptoms were regarded as sexual in origin. Hysteria became a common diagnosis for distress expressed by Victorian women, especially those who did not conform to traditional feminine roles. Gynaecological surgery, including hysterectomy and clitoridectomy, was performed as a treatment for hysteria and insanity. Another strong belief at the time was that work, competition and activity had grave consequences for women's mental health and capacity, so justifying their exclusion from intellectual and employment opportunities.

Freudian theory, for example the concept of penis envy and the notion that the desire for a child is a compensation for lack of a penis, can be seen to reflect the *mores* and attitudes of Victorian society, but, in itself, had a strong influence upon ideas about reproduction and sexuality.

An interesting analogy has been made between the language used to describe production in industrialized societies and the development of medical terminology applied to female reproduction. Emily Martin (1987) noted the emphasis upon production, efficiency, labour and interventionalist control over the reproductive system in medical theories since the 19th century. For example, the doctor can be seen as the supervisor who manages the woman (labourer) who produces the child (the product). Her autonomy and control of the birth are hence diminished.

Twentieth Century Developments

The 20th century has seen the strengthening of medical or biological theories, and advances in medical knowledge. Gynaecology did not emerge as a separate specialty until the early part of this century. Until then general surgeons carried out abdominal surgery for major gynaecological disease, but problems such as menorrhagia, pelvic pain, anaemia and debilitation from repeated pregnancies received little attention. Perhaps because of this historical route gynaecology is still regarded as primarily a branch of surgery.

With increasing sophistication in medical research in the 1920s, the main hormones produced by the ovaries were identified and hormonal treatments began to be developed. During the 1960s the contraceptive pill became widely available, an event which has had tremendous social impact, enabling women to control their fertility. The growth of family planning clinics and well woman clinics in most western societies, has made health care more accessible for many women. Prescriptions for the contraceptive pill peaked in 1976, and fell somewhat later following links with cancer and cardiovascular disease, but this method remains the most popular form of contraception in the UK, followed by sterilization and the condom (sheath).

Developments in oral contraceptives were paralleled, particularly in the USA, by increased prescriptions of hormone replacement therapy (HRT). In 1966 Robert Wilson wrote *Feminine Forever*, advocating HRT or oestrogen therapy for a host of emotional and physical problems. Sales of HRT increased markedly in the 1970s, but subsequently decreased again after studies found an association between unopposed oestrogen and cancer of the womb. HRT is now prescribed with a progestogen (synthetic progesterone) which provides protection for the womb. Initially used as a treatment for hot flushes, HRT is now seen as an important preventative treatment for osteoporosis and cardiovascular disease, which are problems affecting women in later life.

In Britain, childbirth first came under medical management with the advent of six lying-in establishments in London in the 18th century. But most women continued to give birth at home, helped by other women. In 1902 midwives came under state (and medical) control, and in the following years concern with falling population rates focused medical attention on the health of mothers. Initially, hospital confinement was advocated for a small number of high risk mothers; now the majority of first children are born in hospital.

The natural childbirth movements were founded in the 1940s by Grantley Dick-Read in the UK, and by Lamaze, some years later, in France. Popular guides to natural childbirth began to appear in the 1950s. Lamaze encouraged distraction and breathing exercises and later Leboyer drew attention to the environment of the birth, suggesting natural delivery in a dark room. In Britain, the National Childbirth Trust (NCT) teaches psychoprophylaxis and has become synonymous in many people's minds with natural childbirth. Increased technological and interventionist management of childbirth, and the growing prevalence of what is sometimes regarded as unnecessary gynaecological surgery, drew pressure from women's health groups for more control over decisions about their bodies (Phillips and Rakusen, 1978).

In the 1960s and 1970s the women's movement was especially concerned with abortion, contraception and childcare issues. Anxieties about the health risks of the contraceptive pill, diethylstilboestrol (one of the first synthetic oestrogens used for preventing miscarriage as well as other problems) and unopposed oestrogen therapy in the USA led to a distrust of the use of sex hormones. The emergence of self-help groups and alternative remedies began to be explored for a variety of gynaecological symptoms. In the 1980s and 1990s a wide range of support groups has flourished, offering advice and information to women.

The developments in medicine and the parallel growth of alternative or holistic approaches has, to some extent, led to a split between theoretical approaches and practices. People frequently look to conventional medicine for treatment of their physical problems, but emotional and social needs for support, information and understanding are often sought from other settings.

The aim in this book is not to adopt a polarized position, but to enable health care workers and others to combine the best of both approaches. In the next section a biopsychosocial model is described. To redress an existing bias towards biological explanations of illness and health, the influence of psychological and social factors is given particular attention.

A Biopsychosocial Model

The model (see below) represents the many influences (cultural, social, psychological and biological) that can moderate how reproductive changes and problems are experienced and reacted to. The main aim of the model is to attempt to understand the meaning that the problem or reproductive event has for a woman in the context of her life.

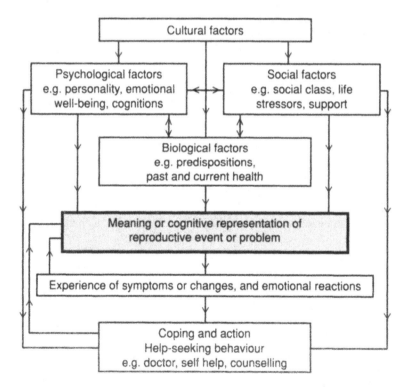

Figure 1.1 A biopsychosocial model of reproductive problems.

This is essentially a model of the woman seeking help. She is seen as actively striving to make sense of her situation. Because her own theories and interpretations are important determinants of her experience, her cognitive appraisal or understanding of the reproductive event or problem is positioned centrally in the model. Although each part of the model is described separately, the interactions between the cultural, social, biological and cognitive factors are also emphasized.

Cognitive factors. Internal thoughts or cognitions include knowledge, attitudes, beliefs, expectations and predictions. When attempting to understand and explain their symptoms, people develop internal representations of their illness: what it means to them, its causes, its duration and prognosis (Leventhal *et al.*, 1980). For example, stomach pains might be interpreted as signifying indigestion or an ulcer depending upon the beliefs, past experience and current situation of the person concerned. People's explanations of symptoms are partly based on available information, and are often influenced by the opinions of those close to them, such as friends and family. Theories are also likely to be affected by a person's general attitudes and beliefs about health and illness.

Understanding an individual's internal representations or model of the problem is important because these perceptions will influence resulting emotional reactions and the extent to which the person seeks medical or other kinds of help. For example, some people tend to use medical labels to describe reproductive changes and look chiefly to doctors for advice, while others might tend to see them as part of normal development and prefer to help themselves or seek non-medical options, such as homoeopathy or acupuncture.

The following cognitive factors have been found to influence the experience of various health problems, as well as help-seeking behaviour:

* Level of knowledge about the problem.
* Explanations of its cause.
* Expectations about the duration of the problem.
* Memories of similar previous experiences.
* The extent to which it is viewed as controllable, by the person herself, as well as by others.
* The value placed on health or reproductive changes compared with other aspects of life.
* Beliefs about her personal ability to overcome the problems.
* Attitudes towards doctors and medical help.

Cultural factors. We have seen how cultural beliefs and traditions influence how problems are expressed and the ways in which they are treated. For example, cultural attitudes towards fertility might have a significant impact on a woman's reactions to hysterectomy. While the operation will have personal meaning for her, in terms of relief from unpleasant menstrual symptoms or disease, cultural values such as the meaning of fertility might also cause her to feel ambivalent about the operation. Culture therefore provides a language or discourse which is drawn upon to create internal representations of health and ill-health.

As suggested in the model, cultural factors can, in addition, have an impact upon social behaviour and lifestyle (for example, diet and family size). These patterns of behaviour and practices can in turn have important effects upon a person's health and well-being. So culture modifies traditions and practices and at the same time influences people's personal perceptions and beliefs. It can have an effect at the social, personal and biological levels.

Social factors. Personal meanings and experiences of symptoms or reproductive changes are closely related to the social context in which they occur. Socioeconomic status, access to employment and childcare, stressful life changes, community facilities, social network and support can all moderate the experience of health problems. For example, a woman with many immediate social difficulties and financial constraints might neglect her own health or delay seeking help. Another person, who might be able to cope with menstrual problems in a supportive social context, may well see them as the last straw if she has no time to rest and constant worries about elderly parents.

Many health variables are associated with socioeconomic status. Health and emotional problems are more common among working class men and women. Working class women are much more likely to experience depression, compared with middle-class women. This finding has been partly explained by the increased prevalence of social pressures on working class women, such as financial and housing problems or stressful life events.

Brown and Harris (1978) carried out a classic study which illustrates how social factors can interact, producing effects which are either beneficial or damaging to a woman's well-being. In a large community study of women living in South London, they found that working class women with two or more preschool children were particularly at risk of becoming depressed when they were faced with a stressful life change (such as moving house, bereavement, accident or divorce). Whether a situation is stressful or not depends to some extent upon the person's appraisal or view of it. Life changes that are seen as uncontrollable, especially losses or bereavements, are common precipitants of depression. In the study, the risks of becoming depressed were raised if the woman had also experienced the loss of a parent in childhood or currently lacked an intimate, confiding relationship. Conversely, rewarding work and close, supportive relationships seemed to act as buffers against stress.

Social factors inevitably impinge upon biology in terms of health risks and health-related behaviours. For example, poverty influences diet, and housing conditions and certain occupations are associated with health problems. Smoking and alcohol, as well as eating, are often used to relieve depression and stress. Smoking has also been found to be a major factor in determining age of menopause, and body fat is an important variable that modifies the level of oestrogen production. In addition, economic factors will, in part, determine access to resources, such as child care, as well as access to health care and choice of treatments.

Psychological factors. Personality and mood affect how changes are regarded and how problems are dealt with. Personality is used here to mean the tendencies a woman has to think, feel and react in certain ways: the way she tends to view herself and the world, and the ways she tends to relate to others. Most people's thoughts, feelings and actions vary considerably depending upon the situation they are in, but particular characteristics can be identified, especially when patterns are repeated over time.

A person's sense of self, and ways of relating to others, is largely learned in early life and develops through subsequent relationships and life experiences. We learn trust, optimism and a belief in our own capacity to deal with problems from early family relationships; from the ways others react to our actions and emotions and from watching how our parents deal with the world themselves. These early relationships affect the way in which we express feelings: how we react to loss, how we deal with physical pain and whether it feels safe to become emotionally close to others.

Subsequent relationships and experiences can provide the opportunity for positive change, while repeated life stresses or unrewarding relationships are likely to be detrimental and might confirm a person's negative view of themselves.

Clearly people have certain predispositions to react in particular ways to stress and to develop psychological problems. There appears to be a genetic predisposition for certain types of severe depression and psychotic conditions, such as manic depression. However, emotional reactions to stress, the extent of these reactions and the form they take also tend to run in families (for example, a tendency to anxiety and worry, often called neuroticism), and these could be partly inherited and partly learned.

How people deal with challenges and problems depends on their mood at the time, but mainly upon their self-esteem. Optimism, a sense of mastery in dealing with the world and confidence in one's own ability, or self-efficacy, are associated with positive adaptation and well-being. Conversely, some people develop a more negative outlook, feeling out of control and pessimistic about their personal effectiveness.

There are, however, specific issues that are relevant to the development of self-esteem in women. Sex role stereotypes and women's second-class status, act as barriers to a positive sense of self. The very qualities that are often encouraged in women, such as being caring and sensitive, are those which tend to be undervalued. In fact, there is a close correspondence between descriptions of 'feminine' characteristics and those deemed 'neurotic'. Attempts to conform to social images or stereotypes of femaleness, frequently mean that women constrain their natural expression of feelings and thoughts and as a result feel dissatisfied, unauthentic or depressed. Women tend to blame themselves rather than acknowledging these social constraints when they feel depressed or frustrated; some may develop physical symptoms such as headaches, or eating problems. Guilt and self-blame are also common following sexual abuse or rape – feelings which often act as barriers to seeking help.

In general, women tend to be judged against 'male' concepts of normality; for example, we are expected to be emotionally stable (meaning in control and consistent), rather than to have moods which are variable, including both highs and lows which are related to the menstrual cycle.

Traditionally, and certainly in most western cultures, a woman's value has been tied closely to her roles in relation to other people, for example, as a mother or wife rather than as an individual in her own right. Moreover, the media presents unrealistic ideals of women as superhuman – attractive, young, perfect mothers, who are successful both inside and outside the home. It is perhaps not surprising that women become disillusioned or disappointed when, for example, the experience of motherhood does not live up to expectations, or when their bodies change as they grow older.

Biological factors. Genetic predispositions to health problems, hormone production, and past history of ill-health can influence how women experience reproductive events or problems. Genetically transmitted diseases, such as thalassaemia and haemophilia, have a considerable impact upon people's decisions about pregnancy and childbirth.

Women with physical disabilities may well experience particular difficulties, for example, during pregnancy and childbirth, especially if the necessary services are not made available. In addition, certain conditions, such as a tendency to miscarry or poorly controlled diabetes, might mean that much of pregnancy is spent in hospital.

Biological predispositions are, however, modified by life experience and lifestyle. For example, a family history of osteoporosis or breast cancer is considered a risk factor for these conditions; but cigarette smoking and reproductive history are also important factors in determining the degree of risk. Current illness and fitness are likely to modify a person's experience of reproductive changes, but these are in turn influenced by social experiences and lifestyle.

Hormonal make-up is frequently seen as a significant factor in 'women's problems'. Although some women appear to be more prone to menstrual problems than others, a particular hormonal basis for premenstrual symptoms or emotional problems experienced during mid-life has not yet been found (Ussher, 1992). Again cultural, social and psychological factors are relevant. Environmental changes, such as diet or stress, can modify hormone production, but more research is needed to understand the role of hormones and their inter-relationships with other variables.

The relative importance of biological and psychosocial factors will depend upon the type of problem experienced. A person's knowledge, beliefs, emotional state and social situation will moderate how symptoms or changes are perceived; in turn, symptoms that are severe and chronic can produce emotional distress and disrupt social relationships and the quality of life.

Emotional reactions and help-seeking behaviour. Let us now return to the centre of the model – the woman's understanding of her problem. This will determine her emotional reactions, the way she copes and the type of help she seeks.

Coping strategies, such as whether to take time off work or whether to attempt to ignore a symptom, will depend in part on expectations about the duration and severity of the problem, as well as on an estimate of her ability to tolerate discomfort. Decisions to seek medical help are also determined by the woman's views of her problem, her knowledge, beliefs and expectations, and her faith in the medical system, as well as her mood and general sense of well-being. Social factors (such as social support, type and availability of medical and other services) are also relevant.

It is important to point out that this model is fluid, in that perceptions of problems are constantly changing, depending upon the input from the various influences described. The woman is viewed here as an active investigator, in that her internal representation of her problem will be modified by new information, discussion and the outcome of her attempts to alleviate it.

In the next chapter a wide range of reproductive events and problems are described, using this broad framework.

Summary

❏ Theories and practices in obstetrics and gynaecology vary between cultures and across time.

❏ Examples from cross-cultural studies show how cultural beliefs and traditions influence how developmental changes and problems are experienced and expressed.

❏ Existing models of reproductive problems – the biological/medical model or the socio-cultural model – fail to adequately represent most women's experiences.

❏ A biopsychosocial model is described which can be used to understand the range of biological, cultural, social and psychological factors which influence women's experiences of reproductive change and problems.

❏ In the model the woman is seen as active in developing her own theories in an attempt to make sense of and alleviate ill-health.

❏ The woman's understanding or internal representation of her problem is central to the model. It is the key influence upon her emotional reactions, coping strategies and the type of help she seeks.

❏ Cultural factors act as a filter through which problems and changes are conceptualized.

❏ Social factors, such as social support, life stress and economic factors, are important influences upon a person's health and well-being, as well as access to services and choices about treatments.

❏ Psychological factors, particularly mood and self-esteem, influence the woman's ability to cope with changes and her ability to pursue solutions confidently.

❏ The woman's internal representations of her problems are constantly evolving as she evaluates the outcomes of her actions and the help she seeks.

2

Experiences of
Reproductive Problems

Empathy, the ability to appreciate and understand another's experience, is one of the keys to effective counselling and communication. To aid this understanding, a broad range of women's experiences of reproductive problems is introduced in this chapter. Women's perceptions of their symptoms and the ways in which they seek medical help are also discussed.

The Perception of Symptoms

'I first thought there was something wrong when one day my period was so heavy that I had to change tampons twice as often as before. You do hear about women having heavier periods in their 40s. When I think about it, they (the periods) have been getting heavier over the last six months.'

(Gail)

'I expected to conceive straight away. I'd had an abortion in my early 20s and thought I must be fertile. It's now nearly a year since we started trying and I feel deep down that there must be something wrong.'

(Jayshree)

'I had had (cervical) smear tests regularly since having the children so I didn't think much about it. When the result came telling me to make an appointment with the doctor because they had found something wrong, I thought there must be an infection – thrush or something – but when he said I had early cancerous changes, I was devastated.'

(Shiona)

The most common symptoms or first signs of reproductive problems are menstrual changes (heavier or irregular periods, spotting in-between periods or no periods), pain and vaginal discharge. Problems can also become evident when expected developments do not take place, as in Jayshree's case, or may be detected by screening programmes, such as prenatal and cervical screening services. Seeing the symptoms or changes as a problem can be a gradual process, as in Gail's example. This insight arises from social comparisons or assessments of what is felt to be normal, as well as from judgements about how tolerable the symptom is, how much day-to-day life is disrupted and how long it is likely to last. In contrast, news of a problem or diagnosis can be received without prior warning signs, as Shiona found.

'My mind became flooded with all sorts of jumbled thoughts, yet at the same time I felt numb and unable to move. Straight away I thought I was going to die. Who will look after my children? Will I have to have surgery, radiotherapy, chemotherapy? How will I tell my family? How did I get this and why me? I had already thought the absolute worst all at the same time.'

Shiona was in no doubt that she needed help, but she was initially extremely upset and confused, as if the problem had been thrust upon her. She had felt healthy prior to this, so the news led to a radical change in her self-concept.

In less acute situations, or when symptoms or changes are mild or moderate, it can be difficult for a woman to know whether her body is functioning normally or not. Symptoms can have quite different meanings depending upon the context in which they occur. Shirley was 47 when she noticed that she was becoming panicky and tense at work. She had already had a spell of anxiety and panic attacks in her late 20s following a divorce, but had recovered from this and was currently unaware of any major stress or change in her life. It transpired that she was having hot flushes, which signified the beginning of her menopause, and which are often associated with palpitations. Because of her history, Shirley had interpreted the palpitations as the return of her old panicky feelings, which led her to feel less in control, and more distressed. Knowledge of the alternative explanation for her bodily reactions helped her to deal with them effectively.

Irregular menstrual bleeding, especially if it is frequent, or occurs between periods, is one of the signs of endometrial cancer (cancer of the womb). If such menstrual changes occur when a woman is in her late 40s or early 50s, they can easily be misinterpreted as one of the first signs of the menopause. This quite plausible interpretation can, however, lead to delay in seeking appropriate medical help.

A woman's perceptions and meanings (or cognitive representation) of a problem will influence how she feels and how she copes with it. People also tend to have learned different ways of coping with problems and their emotional reactions, such as depression, anxiety or irritability, are expressed in various ways. Some people may deal with feelings by talking, crying, complaining, or through activities which help to deal with the problem. Others, and people react differently depending upon the situation, hold feelings inside or bottle them up, which can lead to tiredness, physical tension, headaches, sexual disinterest, sleeplessness or general feelings of unease. Short term relief may be sought via alcohol, cigarettes, drugs or food. Some people feel that it is more acceptable to talk about pain, hormonal changes or physical symptoms than emotional problems.

The way in which a woman makes sense of her symptoms will influence subsequent action taken and partly determine the kind of help received. Interpretations of symptoms can be seen as varying on a continuum from excessive concern and overuse of medical services to total denial of any ill-health. There are cultural differences in the way distress is expressed, and it is important not to judge the physical manifestations of distress as being less valid. Grief reactions following very stressful experiences, such as the loss of a loved one, frequently lead to both physical and emotional symptoms.

Janet, aged 24, came to see a gynaecologist complaining of severe abdominal pain. This occurred for four years, but had become much worse in the past eight months. She had undergone several investigations which failed to find any specific organic pathology and was referred to me, a clinical psychologist, for further exploration of her symptoms. Janet was rather tearful and described how no-one seemed to be able to help her. She had become socially withdrawn and did not feel like doing anything because of the pain. Her primary aim in seeking help was to alleviate the pain so that she could feel better. Discussion of her life revealed that she was a passenger when a close friend, who was driving, died in a road traffic accident. After this event the pain became much worse. Janet felt guilty and blamed herself for not being able to prevent the accident.

'If only I had told her to slow down. I felt as if I knew that the accident was going to happen. I've been so bad since; the pain is so much worse.'

(Janet's story is discussed further in Chapters 4 and 6.)

The Consultation

'It was my first antenatal appointment. I was quite excited because I was going to have a scan as well. I was told I'd see the consultant. But after the long wait

I felt a bit tense. I went in and there was a different doctor. He didn't really look at me and just fired statements at me. After the scan he told me the baby was breech and that I would have to have a Caesarean if it didn't change position and to come back in six weeks. When I got home I just cried.'
(Hansa)

'What I found most difficult was knowing what words to use to tell the doctor about my problem (which was vaginismus). The doctor helped me by talking in more medical words, checking with me and using a diagram. I was very nervous about the internal examination and I was pleased when he told me I wouldn't have to have one at the first visit.' (Sue)

'There was a large room. I went in and there seemed to be so many different people. I felt as if they were all in league and I felt so small. I just wanted to get out of the room as quickly as possible.' (Sally, aged 18)

'I was just so embarrassed when I met the doctor. He was so young and I knew he would examine me.'
(Marjory, aged 62 years, who attended a menopause clinic)

These women's experiences illustrate how distress can result from unmet expectations, problems in communication and anxieties about vaginal examinations. There are several reasons why obstetric and gynaecological consultations are particularly prone to problems with communication and why women's needs for equality, warmth and respect may not be met. The majority of gynaecologists are men, and this makes it more difficult for some women to discuss intimate and personal information. In addition, a vaginal examination is frequently a routine part of an initial consultation.

Only 4 per cent of women surveyed awaiting a gynaecological examination expressed a preference for a male doctor. Forty-two per cent preferred a female doctor, while 54 per cent said that they did not mind either sex (Areskog-Wijma, 1987). They had particular difficulty relating to young male doctors, while older men were seen to be less of a threat because there were less likely to be sexual connotations.

'I've never liked being examined or touching myself. Now you ask, I think it's kind of degrading, as if he (the obstetrician) is seeing a part of me that is embarrassing and distasteful. I suppose I do feel that he can't like doing it either.' (Marjory)

'I don't mind them, I just switch off and think about something else. I pretend my body is not part of me.' (Mary)

One way to deal with anxiety and embarrassment is to distance oneself from the situation as Mary did. Health care workers may have similar feelings of embarrassment and unease and this is often not acknowledged. If they use distancing as a coping strategy, this might confirm a woman's concerns that she is not being treated with care and understanding.

'For me the problem was being talked to with my legs in stirrups while he was examining me. I had no authority or control over the situation; I daren't move. I found myself saying things quite differently than I would have done if I was dressed and sitting talking across a desk.'

Doctor–patient relationships are by definition unequal, since the doctor or health care worker has the advantages of medical knowledge and professional status. However, if symptoms, diagnosis and treatment of problems are discussed during internal examinations, or when the woman is lying down or partially clothed, the power relationship is further tipped towards the professional. As a result of this powerlessness, women might acquiesce to treatment decisions and not express their real feelings and views.

The presence of extraneous people in the examination room is a commonly reported source of unease, especially when their roles are not explained, or the woman's permission is not sought.

'They seemed to drift in and out ignoring me. The doctor spoke to them now and again. The situation made it even harder for me to have my say in what was happening and I felt even more embarrassed and exposed.'

Another woman had a better experience:

'The first time I had a smear test was awful, but this time the nurse explained what was going to happen beforehand. She had a student, but because I was introduced to her it felt better. They also spoke to me during the test, and I had a sheet draped over my legs which certainly helped.'

Aspects of hospital practices and procedures such as long waiting times, block bookings, cramped changing cubicles, being asked to undress before seeing the doctor, and lack of privacy also add to women's dissatisfaction and have a dehumanizing effect.

The problems described so far can not only lead to embarrassment and anxiety, but can also interfere with communication. Good communication can improve patient satisfaction with treatment, facilitate recovery and help prevent unnecessary distress. Unfortunately, communication is often hampered by the professional's use of jargon, failure to properly attend and listen, and lack of adequate explanation and discussion, among other factors.

Mrs B went to see her GP having received a letter indicating 'borderline changes' in her cervical smear test results:

'I had no idea what "borderline" meant, but obviously you think the worst. The doctor said that it wasn't anything to worry about and that I should come back just for a routine check in six months. It was as if that was that and there was nothing else to say.'

Another difficulty arises when the different parties involved hold different expectations or theories about the presenting problem.

'The doctor seemed to be saying that my pain was psychological. How could it be? You can't just create pains. I wasn't convinced. I wasn't imagining it.'

Difficulties in reaching common understandings about problems are more evident when symptoms are non-specific and where there is a lack of medical consensus about their causes. For example, two of the most commonly reported presenting symptoms in gynaecology, menorraghia and pelvic pain, are frequently associated with distress but do not have a known physical cause. Conflicting models are also encountered in discussions of normal reproductive changes such as childbirth and menopause which have been medicalized to differing degrees. Communication during the initial consultation and expectations and theories of both patients and health care workers are discussed further in Chapters 4 and 5.

With the increase in technological procedures for screening and diagnosis, most women will undergo some kind of obstetric or gynaecological intervention during their lifetime. Space does not permit a full discussion of every type of intervention, but a broad range of women's experiences is presented in the remainder of this chapter.

Investigations and Minor Operations

Investigations and minor operations include abortion or termination of pregnancy, D and C (dilation and curettage), cervical cancer screening and sterilization among others. While these are similar in some respects, for example, involving at most brief hospitalization, each clearly has its own meaning. The impact of an investigation or minor operation will depend upon several factors:

- the reasons for the intervention;
- how the decision to undergo the investigation is made;
- expectations of the procedures involved;
- experience of hospital/clinical staff;
- problems occurring during or after the intervention;
- past ability to cope with stressful situations;

- stage of the reproductive cycle;
- the availability of social support;
- the outcome of the investigation or operation and implications for future health.

Experiences of abortion and procedures associated with cervical screening are discussed here.

Abortion or termination of pregnancy

It is now estimated that few serious emotional problems result from abortions or terminations of pregnancy (Donnai *et al.*, 1981) and many women actually report feeling relieved afterwards. However, approximately five to ten per cent of women do have strong, longer lasting emotional reactions, including feelings of anger, loss and regret. Mary (aged 24) and Sophie (aged 36) were unhappy for different reasons:

'I hadn't been terribly reliable with the cap. I actually thought that I might be infertile as I've never been pregnant before. Paul and I have been together for five years and we'd always wanted children. I did have mixed feelings when I found out that I was pregnant. You see I'm in the middle of a training course. It's really important to me. I felt torn in two directions. Paul convinced me in the end, and so did my mother, that it was the right thing not to have the baby now . . . I just felt so confused and superstitious. Will I be able to have a baby later when I want to? I also felt a bit distant from Paul.'

(Mary)

'There were problems right from the beginning. I had two pregnancy tests which gave different results. We decided to have an amnio (amniocentesis) because of my age, and waiting for the result was really difficult. I've always been a worrier. When we had the amnio the doctor assumed that we'd have an abortion if there was an abnormality and we went along with that. I didn't really think there would be anything dreadful wrong but I just felt very anxious. By the time the result came I was 20 weeks. There was a problem (Down's Syndrome) and we went ahead with the abortion. It felt like the best thing. But I didn't realize that it would be like giving birth. The other women in the unit seemed pleased to be getting it over with; I was different and no-one seemed to realize. I felt as if the staff were thinking that it was my fault that I'd left it too late. Yes, that was really the worst part of it.'

(Sophie)

Feeling guilty at such times can increase women's sensitivity to the remarks or behaviour of health care workers. Feeling coerced into the decision, either for or against the abortion, by a partner, relative or doctor, or because of medical reasons, is often followed by regret and confusion. It is worth remembering, however, that in general the outcome is unlikely to be satisfactory for the mother or the child if a woman is refused a termination (Forssman and Thune, 1966).

Cervical screening

Once the most common gynaecological malignancy, cervical cancer has declined in incidence world-wide. The reduction in mortality from cervical cancer in the developed world (an estimated 30 per cent decline between 1960 and 1980) has been attributed to early diagnosis through screening and prompt treatment. However, the efficacy of such programmes has been questioned in the UK, and there is growing concern about the psychological costs of cervical (as well as antenatal) screening (Marteau, 1989).

Large numbers of women in the 1990s are likely to have smear tests, and a proportion will undergo more complex investigations and treatments such as colposcopy or cone biopsy (described below). Common complaints of women undergoing smear tests are the use of confusing terms and definitions, uncertainty and long waits for the results, and not knowing enough about the procedures (Savage *et al.*, 1989).

'I was told I had CIN, abnormal cells and precancerous changes. It was only after I read a lot, saw a diagram and talked to my friend who is a nurse that I got to grips with the whole thing.'

Colposcopy involves an internal examination during which the vagina is held open with a speculum. The cervix is examined using a microscope and samples of the cervix (punch biopsies) may be taken. Cone biopsy is a small operation involving a general anaesthetic, where a cone-shaped piece of the cervix is taken in order to remove abnormal cells.

Posner and Vessey (1988) carried out a detailed study of women's experiences of these procedures. Waiting for the results of the colposcopy or cone biopsy, after having an abnormal smear test result, was identified as the most difficult time by the majority of women in this study.

Many described the colposcopy as uncomfortable, distressing and undignified. They tended to feel anxious beforehand, about the procedure as well as the results, and were very relieved when it was over. The length of time spent lying down in the lithotomy position (the position commonly used for vaginal examinations) with the speculum in place increased their feelings of being exposed and 'clamped, unable to move'. Again embarrassment was experienced especially if their privacy was invaded by extra people in the room. Conversely, staff who talked to them during the procedure, explained what was happening in a 'straightforward' way and who were warm and caring were very much appreciated.

One in four women described the whole procedure as painful: it was the punch biopsies that hurt the most, but again women's reactions varied. As well as the physical pain, it was the idea of an internal, intimate part of them being removed that was threatening. For many the main concern, understandably, was whether they had cancer and what could be done about it.

Cryocautery (freezing treatment) and laser treatment are outpatient procedures that are unfamiliar to most women. The term 'laser' raised some anxieties. Reactions to both procedures were similar. Those women who had not had children were more likely to find the procedures painful or distressing, both physically and emotionally. One in three women said that the procedures were more upsetting than expected. Some had been mistakenly reassured before the treatment that the cervix is insensitive to pain and others were not offered pain relief. Others expected it to take less time. (Cryocautery takes between 10 and 20 minutes, and laser treatment is a quicker procedure.) Veronica explains how she felt after cryocautery:

'When I got home I felt really very shaky, hot and cold. I just wept and had to go to bed. I felt physically and mentally traumatized. I suppose the combination of the worry and what happened at the hospital – having to put a brave face on – got to me in the end. I felt a bit better when I talked to my husband and I've got a friend who's been through a similar thing. The other part of it that I didn't expect was the vaginal discharge (thin and watery) that lasted for about three weeks.'

Those women in the study who had cone biopsy, which involves a three- to five-day stay in hospital in the UK, had more positive responses. Although there were initial concerns about having a general anaesthetic, less pain was experienced and the hospital stay enabled these women to feel cared for.

'It wasn't too bad at all – no housework – time to talk to a great group of other women and being looked after. But seriously it was like a focal point for all those fears and I felt relieved that it's all been taken care of.'

However, others, who had post-operative complications, were less enthusiastic.

Major Surgery

Hysterectomy (removal of the uterus or womb) is one of the most commonly performed operations in gynaecology and for this reason is the main focus of this section. A survey of six European countries indicated that 11.4 per cent of European women had had a hysterectomy. Figures for the United Kingdom were 13.2 per cent and those for France 8.5 per cent (Van Keep *et al.*, 1983). The rate of hysterectomy is increasing and more than twice as many are carried out in the USA and Australia compared to European countries.

Medical decisions to advise hysterectomy are often based on subjective judgements about the seriousness of symptoms. The most common reason for hysterectomy is dysfunctional uterine bleeding, followed by fibroids, pelvic pain and malignant disease.

Recent studies of women both before and after surgery suggest that a woman's emotional state before the hysterectomy is the best predictor of post-operative distress. Many women feel better after the operation, possibly because distressing symptoms, such as severe heavy bleeding, are relieved. Nevertheless, women attending gynaecological clinics and those who have hysterectomies do, on average, report high levels of distress and it remains possible that in some cases surgery is resorted to before other emotional or social problems are adequately explored. The impact of hysterectomy is likely to be determined by the following factors:

* the severity of the pre-operative symptoms;
* age and whether the woman has had children or not;
* circumstances surrounding the decision;
* expectations and beliefs about hysterectomy and its consequences;
* past emotional problems and pre-operative state;
* knowledge about, and preparation for, the operation;
* current relationships and social support;
* surgical approach, for example, vaginal or abdominal;
* whether ovaries were retained or removed.

A young woman, for example, can feel devastated to find that, in order to survive cancer she must give up the thought of having children. Many women express ignorance about what the operation entails. An oophorectomy (removal of the ovaries), carried out at the time of hysterectomy, precipitates menopause and can lead to hot flushes and hormonal changes. The rapid change in hormone levels can make women feel tired and unwell. It is not uncommon for there to be confusion about oophorectomy (removal of the ovaries), hysterectomy or the different implications of these operations.

The following common concerns were voiced when I talked to women pre-operatively.

'I can't afford to be off work for too long. How long will it take to recover?'

I was worried about the pain. Will sex be painful? We have had sexual problems before so I don't want it all to start again.'

'How big will the scar be, will it show?'

'Will I put on weight?'

'I have a small baby and I'm worried about not being able to lift her after the operation.'

As well as worries about the anaesthetic, hospitalization and the emotional and physical consequences of the operation, women were often concerned about the length of time it would take to return to normal life.

Linda is 37, married and mother of a seven-year-old boy, five-year-old twins and an 18-month-old girl. She is healthy and works part-time as a senior administrator. She had already had a vaginal repair operation for a prolapsed womb but her symptoms returned.

'I felt very uncomfortable. It was difficult to put a tampon in and if I ran I leaked (passed water). I'm an active person and I felt very restricted by these symptoms.'

Linda was referred to a consultant gynaecologist who suggested she have a hysterectomy. Although she had expected another repair operation or exercises to be recommended, she decided after much reading and talking to family and friends that a hysterectomy would be the best solution.

'It was an easy decision for me; I've had children, I'll have no contraception or periods. As long as I keep my ovaries it should be fine, and I'm having a vaginal hysterectomy which should be easier.'

Linda wanted to know as much as possible about the operation. She sought advice and read books and leaflets beforehand. She was fortunate to find a 'preparation for hysterectomy' group at a local teaching hospital. So in all respects she would be considered to be healthy, informed and well-prepared. Her main comments about the experiences of hysterectomy are as follows:

'I came to the ward at 4 p.m., the day before the operation. I was assigned a registrar; he was very good. He interviewed me and asked me about the decision to have the operation. He asked me to sign a consent form for the operation and

also, if my ovaries were diseased, to sign for their removal – that was something I wasn't prepared for. He explained that it was very rare and drew a diagram until I was happy I understood everything. I was given a booklet about hysterectomy that night; that was too late really. Luckily I'd read books before coming into hospital. The next day I had suppositories. I was asked to shave my pubic hair completely; if I'd known about that beforehand I'd have felt better. Combined with having suppositories it was demeaning, as if I was abusing my body, doing something I didn't want to do. Apparently I had to shave because I was to have a supra-pubic catheter. I didn't know about this, they didn't really explain, but they were very kind. I had two sleeping tablets and stayed in bed until they took me into the theatre.

I came round feeling very cold. I had morphine for the first couple of days and slept most of the time. I didn't have real pain; I just felt uncomfortable. You're so spaced out you don't feel much. I felt really good at first and relieved it was all over. I was examined on day three. The idea of it was awful; the thought was worse than the experience. In fact it didn't hurt. He (the registrar) was sensitive, kind and considerate.

After three days I felt quite low. I think part of it was the anaesthetic and the operation. I felt a bit weepy. I wanted to go home, I missed the children. I couldn't sleep very well in hospital.'

I asked about recovery and her overall impressions of the operation.

'The recovery . . . it's gone really as I expected. The first two weeks I had to lie down; I couldn't stand much. The difficult part was feeling helpless. I had to rely on my husband, father, friends and neighbours to take and pick up the children from school. It's hard when you're normally fit and active. But the difference each week is encouraging. I feel much stronger now (five weeks post-operatively) and feel as if I'm getting back to normal. Overall, it wasn't too bad, there wasn't really much pain. Now I'm appreciating the positive effects; no symptoms. I think it was important to take what information is available and to seek it out.'

Pauline's experience was different. She is 37 years old and had pelvic pain for seven years. After several operations and treatments for pelvic inflammatory disease she sought help. Pauline has a responsible and pressurizing job. She is divorced and lives with her 20-year-old son. She has a boyfriend who is younger than her and has not had children. I spoke to her six days after her hysterectomy when she was feeling very upset and angry.

'I saw Dr N. twice before coming into hospital and spoke on the phone once. He said the best operation was to have everything removed (womb and ovaries).

He said I should think about it, but I felt as if he'd made up his mind right from the beginning. I didn't want to have my womb removed. The chances of having another child are probably narrow but I might marry again. I'd have liked to have a little longer to try. He said we'll have another chat on Friday. I didn't see him but was given a form to sign. He phoned me later on and I said I didn't want my womb removed; he said something about me being silly. I felt intimidated, I couldn't talk to him. What I felt didn't count.

When I came in for the operation (Saturday), I thought I'd probably lose one tube and ovary, a cleaning up of the pelvis. He came back on Monday evening and explained everything; I'd had the tubes, appendix, womb and part of my bowel removed. I just felt devastated, hard done by, angry and very alone. I feel so different now. I'm still a bit in a vacuum in hospital. I keep thinking about the past, everything that's gone wrong, my marriage . . . I like to be in control . . . I tend to hold back and not let people know how I feel. Since the divorce I've just had to be strong, but last night I asked the nurse to hold me and just cried.'

A week later:

'I've just been going over and over it in my mind. I woke up at 4 a.m. and I can't get back to sleep. It's the choice being taken away . . . a baby – I wouldn't be able to have one now. I see my nephews and nieces. I lie awake. What could it have been like if I'd been able to? It just keeps on, why?'

Pauline faced the operation unprepared, she was pressurized to go ahead with surgery, and was unclear about the extent of the surgery until after the operation. This put her at a considerable disadvantage. In addition, the nature of the operation, as well as the enforced rest from a busy lifestyle, brought her face to face with infertility, her mixed feelings and uncertainties about future relationships, and a deeper feeling of being alone. (Pauline's story will be picked up in Chapters 4 and 6.)

The Experience of Childbirth

'Yes, it was painful but I'd rather be told it's going to hurt for a short time than to have drugs and injections. I think the staff found it hard to let me be in pain. They discouraged me from shouting, and when my husband cried at the end someone said, "What are you crying for?" It made it difficult to express our feelings about our birth.'

'I'd had a Caesarean last time and planned to have one again. It's much easier, you don't have to worry about when it's going to happen and you don't have to go through labour.'

Women's hopes, expectations and experiences of childbirth are greatly variable, but most would not deny the significance of the event and its immediate emotional impact. It brings about a major life change. When anticipating the birth, anxieties about the pain are common, particularly for first-time mothers. The amount of pain reported during childbirth varies considerably between women and from one birth to another, but is described by many as the most intense pain they have ever experienced.

The unfamiliarity of the hospital, the procedures, unexpected events, how one will cope, and the baby's health are common concerns. For many women a major anxiety is about losing control. Noel had two very different experiences:

'With Alex I had a very long labour; 25 hours in hospital, with three different midwives. The difficult thing was to keep going. I think I went in too soon. I had a birthplan and wanted a natural birth. I'd been to classes and used a TENS (transcutaneous nerve stimulation) machine (to relieve the pain). That really worked. But my cervix wasn't dilating and I was very tired. They put in a catheter and I was aware of some problem. I had Pethidine; I was a bit fuzzy. The worst part was when I had the urge to push and they told me not to and left me. I became tearful and discouraged. People were coming in and out for about an hour but didn't interact with me. They could have talked to me and explained more at that time. Alex was born later by ventouse extraction. Afterwards the doctor came to see me on the ward with Alex. That was very nice, it made me feel quite special. I did feel let down after; in the last six to seven hours the control was taken away from me. The support I received at the beginning evaporated later when things started to go wrong. You do feel discouraged, you think you're not doing it right. It's then that you need more support and explanations.

The second time round it was a totally different experience. I stayed at home longer and had a four hour labour and the same midwife throughout. Sally (the midwife) was great. I used the TENS machine and nothing else. It was painful but an exhilarating feeling. I used several positions and I was squatting when he was born. It seems that the staff find it easier to be supportive when things are going well, but it's when you have problems that you need extra attention.'

In a recent study of women in labour, most expected to have more control over their pain and to have fewer medical interventions than they actually had (Slade *et al.*, 1990). The frequency of epidurals, drips to speed labour, monitors, episiotomies and use of forceps all exceeded expectations. Personal satisfaction with labour was strongly related to personal control over it, the ability to control panic and use of breathing exercises. It was unrelated to duration of labour or absolute levels of pain. However, it is not so much a matter of whether technology is used, but whether it is seen to be appropriate, that makes the difference.

There are social and cultural differences in preference for certain procedures and practices during childbirth. However, it is important not to generalize on the basis of social class or ethnic group. Stressing the differences between communities may result in assumptions that a particular group's needs are homogeneous and can readily be identified, which is usually far from true. For example, Asian women are often said not to want fathers present during the birth but, in a recent study, fathers were present at births in large numbers and the couples varied considerably in their needs (Woollett and Dosanjh-Matwala, 1990).

Overall, there is now good evidence to show that women who are socially supported during pregnancy and labour benefit in terms of improved health, both of themselves and their babies (Oakley, 1988). In a recent study of South African mothers, women who were reassured, comforted, encouraged and praised by a volunteer companion during labour, felt that they coped better with the labour, had less pain and anxiety and were more likely to be breast-feeding six weeks after the birth (Hofmeyer *et al.*, 1991). Companionship was thought to reduce the undermining effects of labour in a clinical environment where a woman can feel less competent and in control.

Women's preferences are well expressed in the UK Government Health Committee Report on Maternity Services (HMSO, 1992) which brought together recommendations from individual women, health professionals and community groups. The desire for continuity of care by the same person was emphasized, and midwives were regarded as best placed to provide this. The report concluded that:

There is widespread demand among women for greater choice in the type of maternity care they receive ... many women felt denied access to information which would enable them to make informed choices about their care ... Bad news is given in an unsympathetic way. Too often they experience an unwillingness on the part of professionals to treat them as equal partners in making decisions about the birth of their child. We conclude that until such time as there is more detailed and accurate research about interventions ... women need to be given a choice on the basis of existing intervention rather than having to undergo such interventions as a routine ... The experience of the hospital environment too often deters women from asserting control over their own bodies and too often leaves them feeling that, in retrospect, they have not had the best labour and delivery they had hoped for.

Infertility: Investigations and Treatment

Infertility, the involuntary inability to conceive, is estimated to affect about 10 per cent of couples of child-bearing age, and can result in considerable emotional distress (Pfeffer and Woollett, 1983). In the UK, at least one couple in six can be expected to seek specialist help at some time in their lives, because of an average period of infertility of 2-and-a-half years (Hull *et al.*, 1985). In this same study, the main causes of infertility listed were: problems with ovulation (21 per cent), tubal damage (14 per cent), endometriosis (6 per cent), male problems (26 per cent) and coital factors (6 per cent). Infertility was unexplained in 28 per cent of couples.

Women's responses to infertility vary and they do not follow a unified pattern, but it can deeply affect a woman's feelings of self-worth. Distress is often greatest during the initial medical interview and at the time of diagnosis, and, although reactions understandably differ, most couples experience feelings of loss and grief. Grief over a potential loss is difficult (see page 43) and can embrace feelings of anger, profound sadness, denial, envy, as well as mental preoccupation and physical feelings such as tiredness.

'It took a few hours to sink in that I had a real problem. I felt empty. I can't think about the future at the moment. I just want to cry. Maybe in a few weeks I'll feel better. I just feel deeply damaged.'

Infertility can represent a major crisis that dislodges not only short-term life plans, but also future plans and expectations. Sally had amennorhea for three years after taking the contraceptive pill:

'The treatment (clomiphene) didn't work. I was sent to two other doctors and had a laparoscopy and was given several different diagnoses. The main feeling was of being a failure. As time went on my self-worth became attached to succeeding with the treatment. I didn't use the word "infertility" to describe the problem; it was too painful. In practical terms it was hard to fit in appointments at regular intervals through the cycle when I was receiving a hormonal treatment. I felt as if I had to do it in secret. What helped most in the end was having one doctor who knew my history and was confident and systematic about going through each stage of the investigations and treatment until I eventually became pregnant.'

Guilt and feelings of failure are common and are not helped by common assumptions about fertility. Society expects that married couples will have children, that all couples want children and that it is easy to become pregnant and have children.

'What was terrible for me to deal with was other people's condescending sympathy. They acted as if they could intrude by probing about this intimate aspect of my life, asking why I hadn't got children, and if I did tell them, they just seemed to feel superior to me.'

There is also an assumption that infertility (especially unexplained infertility) is caused by psychological factors or particular personality types. However, attempts to discover particular personality characteristics of infertile women have failed. It is possible that stress might make conception less likely, for example, via increases in prolactin release; but, more research is needed before we can know with any certainty whether and how stress affects fertility. In general, female causes of infertility are overemphasized and male problems relatively neglected.

The need for sex at specified times can lead to sexual difficulties, and expressions of affection and intimacy can easily take second place to the need to perform.

'I found months of taking my temperature and timing sex really wearing. Sex became a chore and it took a lot of effort and talking to avoid blaming each other if it didn't go well.'

Studies of couples' reactions to infertility investigations and treatments in the UK point to unmet needs and gaps in services (Connolly *et al.*, 1987). In particular, these include inadequate provision for the emotional aspects of infertility, not enough information and long waiting times between appointments. Emotional distress was associated with prolonged periods of investigation, and more dissatisfaction was voiced when the cause of infertility lay with the male partner. In one survey of the needs of patients attending an infertility clinic, about one-third said that they would have liked more psychological support and guidance (Edelmann and Connolly, 1987).

The experience of prolonged treatment has been described as a series of hopes and disappointments; plummeting from excitement and joy to sadness and uncertainty (the 'roller coaster ride' of infertility). Such feelings are frequently expressed by women and men going through the new reproductive technological treatments, including in vitro fertilization (IVF), ovum or semen donation (DI), and gametic intrafallopian transfer (GIFT). These are not all widely available, they are expensive, and include a series of investigations and delays before and during treatment.

While bringing fresh hope for some childless people, these treatments entail considerable emotional investment, are costly in terms of time and disruptive to lifestyle. Failure can be experienced at several phases of initial assessment, including egg retrieval (a stage which is described as particularly stressful), fertilization and transfer, and pregnancy testing. The motivation required to persist despite these costs has to be great, given the average success rate which is estimated to be 11.6 per cent (Voluntary Licensing Authority, 1987). It is not surprising that couples tend to overestimate the likelihood of success and experience profound disappointment if pregnancy does not result.

Jo underwent five IVF treatments after being told that her infertility could not be explained.

'It was always successful up to a point. The eggs were fertilized, but the most stressful time was waiting 14 days to see if it had worked. Inevitably you just phoned and spoke to the receptionist who asked if I wanted to book another treatment. You can become really preoccupied. IVF can take over – I've seen it in women. You can't work. You feel so lonely; nothing's happening in your life. I did get depressed . . . In the end we decided to call it a day. We decided to try to adopt. The moment we started to pursue adoption I felt some relief. I suppose I was sick and tired of being prodded about . . . and at the hospital there was a lot of insensitivity and no real continuity of staff. Infertility is not an illness, but the stress is enough to make you ill.'

Jo adopted and now has two children.

Donor insemination can highlight the male partner's disappointment or guilt about his infertility, and brings up particular social and ethical issues as only the biological identity of the female partner is known. The implications of these procedures, such as whether to tell the child, are likely to be increasing concerns for the future.

For some, the continual hope and disappointment can prevent facing the possibility of childlessness and dealing with feelings of loss.

'It was only when I came to terms with life without children and when I could see that I'd really be alright, that life would be different but good in new ways, did I feel better and was able to continue with the treatment in a more confident and less desperate way.'

In a detailed North American study, infertile women identified relationships with a supportive partner, sensitive, supportive friends and sharing experiences with other infertile women, as being of most help to them. Other helpful resources included taking time out to put their problem in perspective, taking advice such as how to apply for adoption, and investing in spheres of life such as work or other children (Woods *et al.*, 1991).

The counselling needs of infertile couples has been recognized in the UK (Human Fertility and Embryology Bill, 1989) with recommendations that centres offering licensed treatment should make proper counselling available to all who require it.

Problems of the Reproductive Cycle

Premenstrual tension, postnatal depression and menopausal problems are described here. Experiences of the different stages of the reproductive cycle vary considerably. For many women, menstruation, pregnancy, childbirth and the menopause present no particular problems. For those who feel tense, anxious or depressed at these times, it can be all too easy to attribute distress to hormone changes. Although hormonal changes obviously do occur, the bulk of recent evidence suggests that, for the majority of women, psychosocial factors (that is, what is going on in their lives) are the most likely cause of distress (see Ussher, 1992, for a review).

Premenstrual tension or syndrome

Premenstrual tension (PMT) or syndrome (PMS) is used to refer to a considerable range of symptoms including tension, depression, irritability, abdominal bloating and breast tenderness (see Warner and Walker, 1992). When asked generally about their menstrual cycles, about 70 per cent of women acknowledge some of these symptoms. However, when PMS is carefully defined in terms of a definite increase in emotional and physical symptoms premenstrually with absence of symptoms in the follicular phase of the cycle, then severe PMS is relatively rare. In an American study, 5 per cent of young women aged 17 to 29 were estimated to have true PMS (McFarlane *et al.*, 1988). This was the case for Vivienne who kept a diary of her moods over a three month period. Although there is some variation between her cycles, a definite pattern emerged.

'I feel like Jekyll and Hyde. Really, you can see my face change. I look drawn and washed out. My stomach is bloated and my moods . . . well I'm just so

sensitive. I cry at the least thing and really can't cope very well with ordinary day-to-day jobs, especially if I have to deal with people.'

For others, ongoing emotional problems can be more difficult to deal with during the premenstrual phase.

'I've always been a bit nervy and I did have a spell of panic attacks and agoraphobia two years ago. I got over it fairly well, but before my period I do feel more tense and irritable than the rest of the time.'

PMS is not a simple biological phenomenon. No consistently abnormal pattern of hormones (oestrogen, progesterone, testosterone, prolactin) has been found, but this does not rule out the possibility of hormonal influences in some women. There is a lot we do not yet know about our reproductive hormones and their interactions. Hormonal treatments (contraceptive pill, oestrogen, progesterone therapy, synthetic progestins) are used, but serve mainly to disrupt the menstrual cycle and have not been found to have any specific treatment effects. Vitamin B6, oil of evening primrose, magnesium and zinc have become popular remedies, and are used by many women, often with beneficial effects. However, there is as yet no conclusive evidence available in their favour from controlled clinical trials.

There is, though, a tendency by both men and women to attribute moods to the menstrual cycle when sometimes other explanations might be more appropriate. For example, women are more likely to attribute the cause of negative events to themselves during the premenstrual phase, but to environmental factors (for example, arguments, problems at work) at other stages of the cycle (Bains and Slade, 1989).

Carol, 26, spoke to Sister J. about her problems at an out-patient clinic. Carol lived alone and felt unable to pursue satisfactory work or training. Since she had left home, she had felt socially isolated, and anxious with other people or when travelling. She said that she felt rejected by her parents.

'They don't really help me. I left home because they were driving me mad, but, look, I haven't made much of a go of it have I? If only this PMT could be treated I'd be able to go to college.'

She frequently returned to the subject of PMT when talking about the unhappy parts of her life. It seemed that by attributing her problems partly to the PMT, she was able to maintain some level of self-esteem. In Chapter 4 we will return to Carol's case.

Postnatal depression

While it is not certain whether postnatal depression (PND) is essentially different from depression in reaction to other life stress, it can be differentiated from the 'maternity blues' and postnatal psychosis. The former is usually described as a transient emotional reaction occurring towards the end of the first week after birth and is estimated to affect 50 to 75 per cent of mothers. The latter is a serious mental illness affecting two per 1,000 new mothers and usually requires psychiatric in-patient treatment. In contrast, postnatal depression affects many women to differing degrees; ten to 15 per cent are estimated to experience severe depression within three months after childbirth.

Psychological reactions to the changes consequent on childbirth, stresses and demands of motherhood, as well as the exacerbation of existing emotional problems, appear to be the main reasons for the increase in depression in women after childbirth. PND has been described as a 'realistic response to the life event of birth and to the stress of maternal role, in combination with other factors' (see Elliott, 1990, and Chalmers and Chalmers, 1986, for a good review).

'Nobody prepares you. They do for labour but not for the baby. You have a rosy picture of motherhood, having a calm baby, but in reality the baby cries a lot of the time. It's exhausting. I walk round the park seeing other mothers being really happy and proud, smiling at their babies. I feel so different.'

'I felt fine for the first week or so then everything started going wrong with the feeding. I wasn't sleeping and the other children were even more demanding. I got really low. It was an effort to take the other children to school. I felt like a wreck, the house was a tip and I just about got the baby and kids dressed and fed. I could see people looking at me and thinking, she can't cope, she's no good as a mum.'

As these examples show, the experience of motherhood, with sleepless nights, tiredness, worries about mothering skills and, possibly, feeding difficulties, can fall far short of idealized media images. After childbirth there is a physical adjustment too; one's body can feel out of control especially when breast-feeding. Some women find that extra weight makes them feel uncomfortable.

'I just worry all the time. The responsibility is enormous. Is she warm enough? Why is she crying? Is she feeding properly? Is that normal?'

It is quite normal to have some of these feelings. Mothering skills, after all, are learned and take practice. But if several problems or anxieties are combined, or if the baby's arrival heralds a dramatic change in lifestyle that is difficult to adjust to, then depression may result.

In a detailed study of 24 women's experiences of childbirth, Paula Nicholson (1990) found that, apart from the physical adjustment and initial insecurities, the degree and quality of support in the early months of mothering was probably the single most crucial factor accounting for emotional distress. Another change that these women had to negotiate was the potential loss of former identity, sometimes including loss of occupation, contacts with friends and colleagues, a social life, and change of role in the family and loss of personal space.

Social pressures can make it difficult to admit to depression. If a mother withdraws and lacks a supportive social network, then depression can become chronic. This, in turn, is likely to affect her relationship with her child and possibly the child's well-being and behaviour. It may lead to marital problems. For single parents, the financial and emotional burden can be still greater, and self-neglect in the interest of the child can increase the likelihood of depression.

The main symptoms of moderate to severe depression are feeling miserable and sad, lacking energy, lacking interest and pleasure in doing things, excessive anxiety and self-doubt, self blame and guilt, as well as physical symptoms such as loss of appetite and early morning wakening (when not caused by the baby!). Again, while some of these feelings may be a common reaction to the stresses of motherhood, if several are present then help should be sought.

The risk of developing postnatal depression is increased in women who experience undue antenatal anxiety, have a family history of psychiatric problems and who have previously had a postnatal depression or psychosis themselves. Previous experience of early loss or of a parent or baby dying during a pregnancy, appears to increase the likelihood of PND.

Problems during the menopause

Hot flushes and night sweats (referred to as vasomotor symptoms) and vaginal dryness are the only two changes (or symptoms) that are specifically associated with the menopause. The menopause, defined as the last menstrual period, occurs on average between 50 and 51 years of age. It takes on average four years from the beginning of menstrual cycle changes to 12 months following the last menstrual period (the definition of having gone through the menopause).

Prospective studies of large general population samples of women from Europe and North America show that for most women the menopause is not a major crisis (see Greene and Visser, 1992). Between 50 and 60 per cent of 45 to 55-year-olds experience hot flushes, and these tend to be viewed as a problem by ten to 20 per cent of women. Approximately two out of five women experience vaginal dryness, which can cause discomfort during intercourse after the menopause. Depression in the average woman is not specifically associated with the menopause. Psychosocial factors such as having negative beliefs about the menopause, being under stress, bereavement, being unemployed and having social problems are the most common predictors of depressed mood, as well as ill-health (Hunter, 1992).

Nevertheless, the range of experiences during this stage of life is considerable and women's reactions to the menopause vary appreciably. For those who find that vasomotor symptoms are problematic, the main reasons tend to be waking at night, and embarrassment and discomfort during the day.

'I just have to throw off the bedclothes several times a night. I'm soaking wet. I have to wash my hair every day and my sleep suffers, so I do get more tired than usual.'

For some women, stress and social attitudes can exacerbate their symptoms:

'I work in a busy office with a few women but mainly younger men. When I get the flushes I do feel embarrassed. I sweat a lot. They are a lot worse in the mornings when there's more pressure on me. Sometimes if I'm talking to someone and a flush starts, I think that the other person is thinking I'm blushing or nervy, you know. I tell close friends and family but I feel that these younger ones wouldn't understand.'

Relaxation can be helpful in relieving hot flushes. Bodily changes, because of their unpredictability, can be difficult to deal with.

'My periods are very irregular now and quite heavy. They were like clockwork before – every four to five weeks. Now one might start when I'm away for the weekend or at work – I just can't tell. My body feels out of control as well with the hot flushes. I don't think they're a real problem. It's just that the changes seem to be using up more of my energy.'

The timing of the menopause is also an issue for some. Premature menopause is roughly defined as menopause occurring before the age of 40, as was the case for Paula.

'Mine came at 34. I had Kay (her daughter) when I was 32 and breast-fed. My periods just didn't start again. I went to see several specialists and in the end they said it was the menopause. I'd never dreamed it could be. I'd wanted another child and was depressed for two to three years really. I had HRT (hormone replacement therapy) and now I do feel better, but it still seems so unfair.'

HRT is often recommended for women who have early menopause, naturally or as a result of surgery (oophorectomy), largely to help protect the bones against the development of osteoporosis.

Clearly the personal meaning of the menopause, whether it heralds infertility as in Paula's example, or represents a relief from periods, or signifies the onset of ageing, will partly determine women's reactions to it.

'I can honestly say I don't mind. It's a natural part of life. I don't feel especially old. OK! I know I'm getting a bit more wrinkled but that's life, isn't it.'

As noted in Chapter 1, myths about the menopause and prejudices towards older women are still pervasive. Negative beliefs can be self-fulfilling. A common belief about the menopause is that it leads to a host of emotional and physical problems, but this is not supported by research findings. It remains possible, however, that some women might be sensitive to rapidly falling levels of oestrogen, as occurs, for example, after surgical menopause (oophorectomy).

Anne came to see me because she felt depressed and lacked confidence. She was having particular difficulties dealing with her teenage son and daughter and had problems with her supervisor at work. Her family's reactions to her menopause seemed to reduce her already low self-esteem.

'They just don't seem to understand. It's got to the stage now that whenever I try to tell them to do anything they think I'm nagging and irritable. It really doesn't help. It just makes me feel more cut off and isolated.'

Anne felt that her attempts at assertion were being put down to 'menopausal moods' and could, therefore, be more easily dismissed.

It is not uncommon for bereavement to be experienced for the first time during midlife, and the emotional and physical reactions to grief may be misunderstood and can, for example, be attributed to menopausal changes. Enabling people to clarify and reach appropriate attributions of distress can be an important part of helping women to deal with this stage of life.

Chronic Reproductive Problems

Pelvic pain

Pelvic pain is one of the most common presenting problems among women attending gynaecological clinics and is often difficult to diagnose. Many women experience long periods of uncertainty and a series of investigations before they feel that their problem is understood. Laparoscopy is usually needed to diagnose conditions such as endometriosis and pelvic inflammatory disease. However, approximately two-thirds of women with pelvic pain are estimated to have no clear pathology following laparoscopy.

'I keep thinking there must be something wrong, especially when the pain is sharp. I know that I've been told there's no actual infection or anything, but when it is bad I am frightened to move about. It really gets me down. People find it hard to be sympathetic when you've got something that doesn't get better.'

Until relatively recently, if no abnormality could be found, the pain was often seen as psychological – 'It's imaginary' or 'It's all in your head'. Pain experienced was thought to bear a direct relationship to the amount of disease or tissue damage. But early theories could not account for individual variations in pain tolerance, nor the increasing evidence that psychological factors such as anxiety, personality and social influences can modify the experience of pain.

In the 1960s Melzack and Wall developed the 'Gate Control Theory of Pain'. This theory proposes that there is not simply a one-to-one relationship between physical damage and experience of pain. Pain messages are modulated by descending influences from the brain. The gate, an integrating mechanism at spinal cord level, balances this input from the brain (including attention, mood and past experience) with peripheral input, such as a pinprick. This balance opens or closes the gate to transmission of pain messages, making a person more or less sensitive to the pain (see Melzack and Wall, 1982).

The gate control model is a helpful way of thinking about chronic pain. As it becomes more chronic, the influences of attitudes and behavioural reactions to pain become more relevant. The model has the advantage of invalidating the dichotomy betwen real or organic pain and imaginary or psychogenic pain. Thus all pain is seen as real, but the factors maintaining pain may vary. Even when physical causes are identified, a person's mood and reactions to the pain will affect the way it is experienced.

Despite these advances in understanding, women with unexplained pelvic pain are still sometimes described, usually pejoratively, as having conflicts about sexuality or femininity, or as 'hysterical' personalities. Endometriosis and pelvic inflammatory disease are common causes of acute and chronic pelvic pain. Endometriosis affects between one and two per cent of women. It is the second most common gynaecological disorder after fibroids. It is diagnosed in about 25 per cent of operations, and causes pain and in some cases infertility. It is defined as the presence of functioning endometrial tissue outside the uterine cavity but its precise aetiology is unknown. Hormonal treatments can provide relief from symptoms, but it is estimated that up to two-thirds of women will have a recurrence after most treatments. Surgery is often the only choice offered in severe cases. The endometriosis sufferer has been stereotyped as being white, middle-class, middle-aged and female and endometriosis has been labelled as a career woman's disease, but there is no strong evidence to support such views. In fact the condition has been found to occur throughout the childbearing years.

In a survey of over 700 of its members in the UK, the Endometriosis Society found that a considerable time lag between the onset of symptoms and a definite diagnosis was a commonly voiced concern. Women also had difficulties in communicating their symptoms to health professionals. There were confusions about what is a normal part of being a woman and fears that discussing certain symptoms leads to being labelled neurotic (Hawkridge, 1987).

If severe and chronic, endometriosis can have an appreciably negative impact upon emotional well-being and quality of life. Chronic pain commonly leads to tiredness and depression, and the impact of endometriosis on sexual relationships and fertility can put strains upon relationships and limit future life plans.

Pelvic inflammatory disease (PID) refers to infection and inflammation of the pelvic organs and is caused by bacteria or viruses. Infection enters the pelvis via the cervix and spreads along epithelial linings of the uterus and tubes. If not diagnosed and treated early, the infection spreads to the supporting structures and causes adhesions. It can be acute, chronic or recurrent, and symptoms vary, but pain in the lower abdomen is the main symptom. The pain is often worse on one side and may occur during intercourse, menstruation or ovulation and may be intermittent or constant. In view of the variation in pain characteristics and other symptoms (such as nausea, fatigue, fever, bleeding), PID is difficult to diagnose conclusively other than by laparoscopy. Treatment for acute episodes involves antibiotics and complete rest. If treatment is delayed and the condition becomes chronic, it is usually more difficult to treat. Fertility can be affected and adhesions and scar tissue can add to the pain.

Gynaecological cancer

Cancer evokes strong feelings of fear and dread in most people. Intense depression and confusion are common reactions to a diagnosis of cancer. These feelings are not surprising given the frequent difficulty in locating a cause, uncertainty about the prognosis of the disease, the side effects often associated with treatment and the long-term psychological and social implications. For example, there are usually worries about the impact of cancer upon one's future and the lives of family and friends. Fears of enduring a painful and undignified death are also common. For a detailed overview of the impact of cancer and the effects of treatment, see Fallowfield (1991).

The most common site for gynaecological cancer is the endometrium (womb) which occurs mainly in peri- and post-menopausal women. This is followed by cancer of the cervix, the ovary and the vulva. Gynaecological cancer can bring additional specific concerns including the effects of gynaecological surgery and treatment upon fertility, sexual functioning and self-image. Sheila had a smear test and was sent immediately to a hospital for an examination, where she was told that she had cancer of the cervix.

'After the doctor told me, I was stunned and cried for nearly an hour in the sister's office. It was not being able to have children that really brought on the tears; the option gone in one fell swoop.'

Sheila is divorced with a teenage son and has had a four-year relationship with her current partner.

'I had to alter my whole way of looking at my future. That was the first reaction – no children. Survival was secondary at that point.'

For some women the idea of cancer is especially disturbing. In one survey, women described cancer in metaphorical and very negative terms as an unstoppable destruction of the human being and spirit (Posner and Vessey, 1988). The association of some gynaecological cancers in popular literature with past sexual experiences and the contraceptive pill can increase self-blame and guilt. Lack of adequate information often compounds the situation. While most doctors now believe that patients should be told that they have cancer, patients frequently remain inadequately informed about their illness and of the treatments they face.

Treatments for cancer can be unpleasant. Nausea and vomiting, hair loss, lowered energy and appetite are often reported after chemotherapy. Radiotherapy can produce skin irritation, lethargy, nausea, as well as ovarian dysfunction. Menopausal symptoms and infertility result from irradiation of the ovaries.

Radical surgery is sometimes necessary. Ivy underwent a vulvectomy to treat cancer of the vulva. Not surprisingly this operation can be extremely difficult to adjust to and leads to major sexual difficulties in 70 to 90 per cent of women.

I was very bad for months. It was hard to look at myself and sex was not possible the way I felt. Harry was so good. In the hospital the nurse was so kind; she helped me to look, and, because she wasn't shocked it made me feel less ashamed. I know it will take time, but I don't think I'll ever feel the same as I did. I'm glad to be alive though. When you've been through what I've been through you see what's important in life.'

Following a period of intense investigation and treatment, going home, often with an inevitably vague prognosis, can be very difficult to deal with, and includes dealing with other people's reactions as well as one's own. As Sheila remembers:

'You have to do something different. I found healing helpful. I really needed it to help the panics. I had lots of good friends, read lots of self-help books. I did everything. I met lots of people who gave me different outlooks. I think it's too much for one person (her partner) to bear. You're so needy; one person isn't enough; you have to get help elsewhere as well. I didn't want to be treated with kid gloves. It helped to use the word cancer – the more you use a frightening word the less frightening it becomes. I realized that my reaction dictated other people's reactions. If I was strong other people could deal with it and were more positive.'

Bereavement and Pregnancy Loss

'The death of a baby, whether at birth or in the weeks or months immediately afterwards, is no less a death than any other . . . It is certainly different, but it is not a lesser event.'   (Kohner and Henley, 1991)

The term pregnancy loss is used here to include miscarriage (loss of baby before the 28th week), stillbirth (a baby born dead after 24 weeks), and neonatal death (a death occurring within 28 days after birth), as well as loss of a baby due to abortion for fetal abnormality. While these experiences are different, it is now generally acknowledged that grief is a common and natural reaction following the loss of a baby at any stage. A baby's death is the loss of a person who would have been. This can mean the loss of a new identity as parents and the loss of dreams and future plans.

Although there are huge individual differences in the way people deal with loss and bereavement, there does seem to be a typical pattern to the grieving process. Typical grief involves three main stages (which may not always be experienced in this order):

• An initial reaction of numbness or denial, which usually lasts two to three days.
• A second stage of despair or full grief reaction, which varies in duration and intensity. It is often experienced with feelings of sadness, depression, anger, guilt and self-reproach, as well as withdrawal and reduced contact with others. This is a painful stage which often entails dealing with conflicting feelings.
• In the third phase of recovery, life is gradually adapted and rebuilt to accommodate the changes needed in response to the loss. (For detailed accounts see Parkes, 1978.)

The length of time this process takes varies greatly depending upon the relationship with the deceased, as well as previous experience of loss, ability to cope, social support, cultural factors and the circumstances surrounding the death. Grief may be felt to be lifting when it is possible to think of the deceased person without the painful wrenching quality experienced earlier, though of course, a sense of sadness inevitably persists.

Four main tasks of grief have been identified:

• To accept the reality of the loss; it is often difficult to believe its finality.
• To experience the pain of grief. Denial or excessive avoidance of emotional reactions, by pushing them away or keeping busy, can prevent healthy resolution of grief.
• To adjust to an environment in which the deceased person is missing.
• To withdraw emotional energy and reinvest it in another relationship or activity.

Providing support after pregnancy loss is discussed in more detail in Chapter 5.

Miscarriage

Miscarriage is not an uncommon event. Up to 20 per cent of all pregnancies end in miscarriage before 20 weeks. It is often assumed that during the first trimester a woman is unlikely to have become attached to the pregnancy. However, many women do think of the fetus as a real person and seeing the baby on an ultrasound scan can reinforce this feeling. Bonding and attachment to the unborn child, for many women, begins during pregnancy.

'I was 14 weeks pregnant and looking forward to my first scan. It seemed to take a long while for the radiographer to find the heart beat. I was oblivious really. Looking back he might have been trying to tell me, I think, but I didn't take it in; I just thought it was the equipment. But when we went back to see the doctor he told us the baby had been dead for some time. It was terrible, I'd been so happy. For weeks after, I couldn't concentrate on work and I kept crying at home. They told me that the baby wouldn't have been normal. That was supposed to reassure me but it made me feel worse. Not only had I lost a baby but I'd even produced an abnormal one!'

Such feelings are not uncommon amongst women experiencing miscarriage in early pregnancy. In a British survey, women appreciated doctors who discussed their distress and grief, and were generally angry to be told that it was only an early pregnancy and that they should try again. They also felt that they were given conflicting advice about how long to wait before trying to conceive. In general, the women tended to view their miscarriage as a serious loss, while from the doctors' perspective it was a common clinical problem (Friedman, 1989).

Abortion following fetal abnormality

With the increasing use of sophisticated techniques of prenatal screening and diagnosis, the number of pregnancies terminated for fetal abnormality can be expected to rise. The majority of abortions carried out for fetal abnormality are terminations of wanted pregnancies. They are usually carried out in the second trimester which means inducing labour – an experience which can be very distressing. Even when the baby would not have survived, many women feel guilty about having made the decision to end the baby's life. There is also the additional anxiety about whether the abnormality will recur in future pregnancies.

Stillbirth, perinatal death and neonatal death in first week of life

There are approximately eight perinatal deaths (which include stillbirths and deaths in the first week) for every 1,000 live births in England and Wales (OPCS, 1990). Sometimes there are warning signs indicating that something is wrong, but frequently the parents learn of their loss at birth or shortly afterwards.

Stillbirth has, in the past, been viewed as a non-event. There was little expectation of grief, and parents were encouraged to forget about it and have another baby. Since the late 1960s, with the pioneering work of Bourne and Lewis and others, the feelings and needs of bereaved parents have been taken seriously, and considerable steps have been made in the 1980s to improve health care and voluntary services for couples who have lost a baby (see Kohner and Henley, 1991).

Strong grief reactions are normal and common following stillbirth and perinatal death. Parents usually develop strong feelings towards a baby before the baby is born. But parents who have a stillborn child or who lose a child shortly after birth face particular difficulties. It is bewildering when expectations of a joyous birth are swept away and instead the parents are confronted directly, often for the first time, with death. As Naz described:

'A tragic thing has happened to us yet as far as everyone else is concerned there is nothing to see. I know that baby, he was part of me and he has died. I want to tell the world about how unfair it is, but no-one finds it easy to talk about death. The whole thing feels unreal. It's nearly three months now, but I still dream that all this hasn't happened, and I can somehow be pregnant again and have another chance.'

This feeling of confusion is very common. Having no tangible object to mourn presents difficulties in dealing with feelings during the first stage of grief which involves accepting the reality of the loss. Feelings of unreality can be greater if an epidural for labour or a general anaesthetic for delivery was used, and the situation is still more confusing if the imagined perfect baby was found to be malformed in some way. In addition, there is often a 'conspiracy of silence' surrounding the death, with people wanting to avoid talking about the loss because of awkwardness and embarrassment. There may be less bewilderment if the baby survives longer because the couple have had direct contact with life and death.

Sensitive handling at the time of loss includes enabling the couple to have time to hold the dead baby, to have a photograph or some other memento, and a funeral. (In Britain, a funeral is arranged if the baby is born live or is stillborn after 24 weeks, but it is possible to arrange a burial for a baby stillborn before 24 weeks if the parents so wish.) These events can all help to mark the experience and to provide a focus for grief.

Understandably parents want to know why their baby died. Anger is a normal part of grief, but if no clear cause of death is evident, anger may well be expressed within the family, towards friends or against the hospital. Guilt and self-blame can lead to increased sensitivity, which in turn interferes with closeness and support which is needed at this time. Parents may go through the stages of grief at different rates and have different ways of expressing their feelings. There are ample opportunities for misunderstanding. Naz describes the effects of her loss on her relationship with her husband, Tariq.

'I suppose I do think it must have been something I did during pregnancy or maybe my genetic make-up. I cry a lot and really want Tariq to reassure me but I suppose I ask indirectly and too often and he finds it hard when I cry. He deals with it differently; he goes quiet . . . I know he's thinking about it, but he doesn't want to talk in case I cry.'

Other common reactions include avoidance of the hospital and other people who have babies. The intensity of mixed feelings can be hard to tolerate. Jen's baby died two days after birth seven months ago.

'I can only look at the photo when I am with Dave at home. If I go out and see anything that triggers me off, I try to avoid it, because I know that if I start to cry the feelings might get out of control. At times I feel as if I'll explode or go mad.'

(Jen's story will be explored further in Chapters 4 and 6.)

Some parents will find that grief is more difficult to deal with than others. An early loss in childhood or early emotional deprivation appears to diminish a person's capacity to deal with loss. Similarly those who have had previous emotional or psychiatric problems and a previous pregnancy loss may find grief more difficult to bear. Women who had strong, mixed feelings towards the pregnancy or who initially did not want to have a baby, may experience greater guilt and find grief harder to resolve. The loss of a twin or multiple birth can complicate the grief process, because to experience both loss and joy is inevitably difficult. Couples in this situation might need help to separate their feelings about the dead child from those towards the surviving child or children.

Long-term consequences of unresolved grief can include persistent denial of the loss, excessive and long-lasting self-blame, guilt and depression. Grief may also re-emerge in later life following another loss. Social support is helpful, and a good intimate relationship is highly valued. However, recent attention has emphasized the appreciable benefits that can be achieved for grieving couples, if the situation surrounding the loss is managed well (see page 99).

Summary

❏ Women's experiences of reproductive changes and problems vary considerably. Their impact depends upon the individual significance of the change or illness, its nature, and the psychosocial context.

❏ Women frequently voice many concerns about their treatment in obstetrics and gynaecological settings.

❏ Talking about intimate aspects of their lives and having vaginal examinations are sources of anxiety.

❏ Women, in these settings, often feel misunderstood and are dissatisfied because of poor communication and lack of opportunity to discuss problems fully.

❏ They value clear information, the opportunity to be involved in decision-making, and some control over their treatment.

❏ They want to be informed about the logical stages of treatment and what they can reasonably expect to happen.

❏ They feel helped by people who show concern and understanding and who listen; these qualities are particularly needed when normal procedures go wrong, or when women feel especially vulnerable or unwell.

❏ Practical and procedural aspects of health care are especially distressing. These include long waiting times, inadequate changing facilities, lack of follow-up appointments and seeing different staff at each appointment.

❏ Social support is generally felt to be of benefit, whether from a partner, family, support groups or health professionals.

❏ Some women need someone to listen, to help them to clarify the causes of their symptoms or feelings, and time to think about how to deal with emotional, health or life problems.

❏ Women or couples dealing with loss or chronic ill-health face the emotive issues of receiving bad news and coping with feelings of grief.

3

Counselling:
Definitions, Aims, Process

Opinions vary appreciably as to what exactly counselling is, what it should be and who should do it. Nevertheless, most people would agree that communication skills are fundamental to all interactions with people, whether they are seeking help or working with colleagues. Such skills include listening, exploring and clarifying problems, giving advice and information, as well as support. In contrast, formal counselling is carried out by health care workers and others who have special training and regular supervision. The British Association of Counselling defines counselling as follows:

> An interaction in which one person offers another person time, attention, and respect, with the intention of helping that person explore, discover and clarify ways of living more successfully and toward greater well-being.

MacLeod Clark and colleagues (1991), who are nurse counsellors, describe a hierarchical model in which communication skills can be built upon and developed, with training and supervision, into counselling skills. Counselling skills include empathy, genuineness, being non-judgemental, setting goals, and supporting and challenging. The use of counselling skills is distinguished from formal counselling which requires specific training.

A broad definition of counselling will be adopted here to include most interactions between health care and voluntary workers and women or couples seeking help, as well as settings in which counselling is arranged on a more formal basis. The term counsellor will be reserved for those employed professionally, and who have a recognized training, while the term helper will be used to include anyone in contact with people in a helping role, whether working in a statutory or voluntary health care setting.

Aims of Counselling

Two broad aims of counselling will be addressed:

1. To meet the needs, expressed by women in the preceding chapter, for good communication, provision of adequate information, and emotional support.
2. To be able to offer specific kinds of help for those with particular issues, such as women faced with difficult decisions, those who are distressed, or those who need help to clarify problems or to come to terms with ill-health.

It is hoped that the communication and counselling skills described in this and the following chapters will provide guidelines applicable to a variety of situations. For example, these might range from discussions about contraception at a family planning clinic, or a health visitor talking about coping with a new baby, to counselling prior to an abortion or fertility treatment, to giving bad news about a pregnancy or a screening result. In addition, the same skills may be used to help women and/or couples to clarify their own difficulties, and to support them in dealing with loss or chronic health or life problems.

Different levels of counselling are appropriate depending upon the situation, the skills, the expertise and role of the health care worker, and the expectations and needs of the person seeking help. Nevertheless, good communication skills, the basis of all counselling, are desirable in all settings and, if practised, yield benefits for all concerned.

Clearly counselling, as defined here, cuts across professional boundaries, but it is important to acknowledge one's own level of training and skills. This book cannot hope to provide training in counselling (for counselling courses, see page 133), but it does offer practical examples of ways of improving existing skills and making these sensitive to the specific needs of people seeking help in obstetrics and gynaecology. Some individuals seem better than others at communicating, but these are skills that can be learnt and are best maintained by staff support and training (see Chapter 7).

The Relationship: Expert or Helper?

The counsellor's role is to facilitate the client's work in ways that respect the client's values, personal resources and capacity for self determination.

(British Association of Counselling, 1989)

This description suggests a degree of equality and mutual participation in the counselling process. It contrasts with the traditional role of the health care worker (typically doctor) as expert, testing his/her theories and prescribing advice and treatment with little concern for the patient's perspectives. Three types of doctor–patient relationships have been described by Szasz and Hollender (1956), which vary according to the patient's feelings of autonomy and level of participation:

The activity–passivity relationship. Here, as implied, the doctor/helper is in charge and the patient is passive, does not participate and is expected to accept decisions that are made. This relationship may be appropriate in certain emergency situations, but is counterproductive when the aim is to understand the patient's problem.

The guidance–cooperation relationship. In this relationship the patient is offered some autonomy and participates more, but the terms of the relationship and the agenda of the discussion are laid down by the doctor/helper. This expert role of the health care worker is often reinforced and maintained by people's expectations and hopes that someone will solve all their problems. In some situations this model is appropriate, for example, when people are extremely ill. However, the negative outcomes of this type of relationship are that people's theories may not be explored fully and they may not express their concerns and opinions. This way of working leads to many of the dissatisfactions expressed by women in the previous chapter.

The mutual participation relationship. This is usually the most desirable relationship for helper–patient interactions. Here the assumption is that both participants are active and exercise personal responsibility for the content of the interaction and its outcome. Obviously differences exist in terms of professional status, but these can be acknowledged and the aims of mutual participation made explicit. Seeking out the patient's views, expectations and opinions helps to maintain this cooperative relationship.

Another way of describing these relationships is in terms, used in transactional analysis (Harris, 1967), of parent, adult and child interactions. The expert model (or guidance–cooperation relationship) is similar to a parent–child interaction, whereas the optimal counselling relationship involves adult–adult interactions. By assuming a parental role one tends to position the other person in the child role; a situation which is often encouraged by the setting (for example, if the person is lying down, feeling unwell and vulnerable). Conversely, by engaging in 'adult' conversation, one addresses the patient as an adult, as someone who can take responsibility for themselves. This mutual participation or adult–adult model is similar to that described by Egan (1990). He views the counselling relationship as a collaborative process between helper and person seeking help. His approach provides a general framework for helping people to help themselves and is described more fully in the next section.

The Counselling Process

This book cannot attempt to provide a comprehensive description of the array of available counselling models and psychological theories, although Nelson-Jones (1988) gives detailed discussions of a variety of different models.

Many people develop their own counselling style; an eclectic approach drawn from different theories. The model of helping described here is derived to a large extent from Gerard Egan's (1990) problem-management approach. This is an eclectic model which is practical and skills-based. The clear framework of this model is particularly helpful for training others and for those who wish to improve their counselling skills. In addition, his approach, together with ideas from client-centred therapy (Rogers, 1961) and social learning and cognitive theories, is consistent with the biopsychosocial model of the person seeking help (see Chapter 1). The author's own work, and the counselling approach outlined here, is also influenced by feminist thinking (see Eichenbaum and Orbach, 1983, and Chaplin, 1988, for examples of feminist approaches).

Carl Rogers has perhaps had most influence upon counselling practice. His client-centred or non-directive approach is appealing because it focuses upon the individual's inherent tendency towards self-regulation. By asking open questions and listening carefully, the helper begins by encouraging the person to tell his/her own story. Central to his theory is the importance of the person's self-concept (the ways in which individuals see and define themselves) and positive adaptation. The individual is respected and is regarded as responsible for his/her own development. However, positive change is facilitated by a certain type of helping relationship.

Rogers strongly maintained that empathy, respect and genuineness in the helper constituted the 'necessary and sufficient conditions of therapeutic personality change'. These are fundamental attitudes that are crucial for good communication and counselling in health care and other settings.

Empathy refers to the attempt to enter the private world of the other person and to perceive the other's point of view accurately. The helper tries to be sensitive to the person's understandings, feelings and experiences and attempts to communicate this awareness to him/her. It will not be possible to understand someone else totally, and some people may be more difficult to empathize with than others. However, the task is to try to reach a fairly accurate view of the other person's model (or cognitive representation) of their problem. You may not agree with their beliefs or theories, but the very process of attempting to clarify the person's internal thoughts and feelings can make them feel valued, as well as providing the groundwork for discussion of different ways of looking at problems.

Respect means valuing and accepting the person for themselves. It involves not judging people or assuming a superior role, but taking care to listen. The knowledge, experience and views of the person are appreciated, taken seriously, and given equal (if not more) weight when compared with 'expert' opinions. If respected, people are more likely to feel responsible for their health and decisions, more actively involved in treatment, more likely to value themselves and more able to help themselves.

Genuineness suggests a number of qualities, including honesty and integrity in relation to the person seeking help. It also implies being honest about one's own shortcomings, such as biases or prejudices, and being able to admit lack of knowledge or skills. Being genuine means being truly interested in helping someone, and is conveyed to the person by politeness and reliability, by attention and listening, and by maintaining confidentiality.

There is some overlap between these fundamental attitudes and how they are communicated; together they help to build a relationship of trust. If people are shown empathy, respect and genuineness then they will learn to value themselves, be less defensive and be more effective in solving their own problems. It is worth emphasizing here that, although these qualities are often discussed within the context of formal or professional counselling, I believe that these can be achieved, and should be attempted, in all meetings with patients (see Chapter 4).

Egan describes the counselling process in three main stages:

1. The problem is explored and clarified, as well as the person's internal representations (or models) of it.
2. A common understanding of the problem is reached and goals are agreed upon and set.
3. Changes are implemented using a problem-solving approach. The impact of change is then evaluated and fed back to inform the initial understanding of the problem.

It may not seem appropriate to progress through all these stages with every patient, but this framework is really a way of evaluating hypotheses about the problem with the person seeking help, and therefore is relevant to most patient–helper interactions, however brief. For example, in discussing what type of contraception a woman might choose, it is important to explore her views, her past experiences and her ideas about the appropriateness of a new regime. Based on this information, as well as medical knowledge, a decision is taken. At a subsequent meeting the suitability of the method and its effectiveness can be discussed with changes made if necessary.

This approach offers a synthesis of ways to help people to find solutions to their own difficulties. The helper is usually non-directive, but also participates, at times by offering information, suggestions and alternative perspectives. The problem itself and the goals of counselling are clearly defined at the beginning, and the responsibilities of both the person seeking help and the helper are made explicit.

Clarifying the problem

Here the aim is to help the woman to identify, explore and understand her problem. The helper at this stage generally asks open questions (see page 69) and follows the woman's story, seeking clarification where necessary. A positive and supportive relationship is established, ideally by the helper showing the qualities of genuineness, spontaneity and openness. In this setting, a woman will feel freer to explore her problems and not feel obliged to present only one side of her story. By careful attention to her words, tone of voice and behaviour, the helper is more likely to be able to understand and to feed back that understanding (that is, show empathy). This is often a gradual process of checking back with the person to make sure that you are not misunderstanding.

When initially seeking help, and especially if feeling unwell, it is not unusual for women to feel more passive and depressed than they normally would. They might feel embarrassed about asking for help, or uncomfortable about appearing weak and vulnerable. Such mood states are likely to render a woman more sensitive to the feeling that the experts know best and make her less confident about expressing her own opinions. There may well be issues that are difficult to talk about such as sexual abuse or rape. It is also common to become more sensitive to criticism when feeling low. The health care worker will need to communicate understanding to the woman in order to help her to feel comfortable and to feel able to talk about problems in her own time.

As well as facts about events and symptoms, it is important to gain a broad impression of the woman's current thoughts, feelings and behaviour. Her theories about the causes of her problems can be explored, as well as her future expectations and her beliefs about her own ability to overcome her problems.

The biopsychosocial model (see page 9) can serve as a working model for the helper in order to think about the range of possible influences upon the person and her problems. These may include the personal meaning of her symptoms or problems, their impact, but also the psychosocial context in which they occur, for example, what was going on in her life, how stressful a life change is, and how she tends to cope with problems generally.

It is clearly best to begin by hearing and following the woman's story and her understanding of it, and then to examine the implications of her theories and beliefs. One of the most important things that helpers can do is to take time to discuss different ways of looking at a problem with the aim of identifying new, more useful perspectives. Alternative explanations of problems can be discussed in a tentative way. Part of the helper's role might be to offer information. It is often useful to make explicit the assumption that there are usually various ways of conceptualizing a problem, some being more helpful than others. Both people can then work together to identify key issues and discuss likely explanations and the implications of these.

When discussing problems and models, you will hear how the woman thinks about herself and her life in general. She might reveal how she thinks she should behave or look or feel. She might assume that there is one physical cause for all her problems, or she might tend to describe most people in her life as unhelpful. Methods used in cognitive therapy can be used to examine the validity of some of these beliefs or assumptions. These include the identification of thoughts that are repeated in the woman's descriptions and enabling her to think about more complex explanatory models.

Depressed people have been found to engage in what might be described as self-defeating thoughts. When depressed, we are more likely to attribute the cause of positive events to other people and the cause of negative events to ourselves. When not depressed we tend to do the opposite and to be more optimistic about ourselves and our achievements. For example, two people might be told they did well at a project at work. One might say, 'Oh well, anyone could have done that – it was easy'; while another, by saying 'My work is going well, I must be good at my job', increases their own sense of self-worth. The helper in this situation can usefully encourage a woman to become aware of such patterns in her thinking.

Much distress results from people's internal constraints, or their beliefs and expectations about themselves. Women, in particular, internalize social expectations that they *should* be thin, caring, sexy or attractive, and as a result attempt to exert often unrealistic controls over their feelings and behaviour, for example, by dieting or by being overly self-critical. Some women experience inevitable feelings of failure in the attempt to be a 'perfect' mother, daughter or wife. Another common belief is the idea that one does not deserve help, or that the needs of others should always come first. Guilt and anxiety, resulting from conflict between internal constraints and natural desires, are not uncommon; for example, from the realization that living to please others does not satisfy one's own basic needs. Pointing out and questioning these internalized social attitudes can be liberating; more realistic ideas and expectations about the person can then be explored.

One woman, I will call her Sue, came to see me because she was distressed because she had experienced her menopause two years previously, when she was thirty. Exploration of the personal impact of this event revealed that she had felt considerable sadness and disappointment about the effects of menopause upon her fertility. However, she also felt that she had aged and that there was little point planning for the future. It became clear that she believed that menopause meant that she would rapidly age and become unattractive (a common stereotype in western cultures, see page 5). I provided some information about menopause and discussed her emotional reactions to infertility, which had become less intense over time. By voicing her fears, she separated the issue of fertility from a more global, negative reaction to the menopause. After much discussion, a shared understanding was reached that she was grieving her loss of fertility, but that her self-esteem had suffered, in addition, from beliefs about the menopause which were overly negative. This shift in her appraisal of the problems enabled her to begin to think more positively about herself and her future.

Cognitive therapy is a method of helping people to examine their internal representations of themselves and their problems. People are encouraged to challenge unhelpful assumptions, as outlined above, and to look at the effects of these thoughts upon their feelings and behaviour. For detailed accounts of cognitive behaviour therapy, see Dryden and Trower (1988); Hawton et al. (1989). For an excellent but more complex analysis of cognitive psychotherapy Brewin (1990) is recommended.

As well as examining cognitive constructions of problems and events, it is important not to overlook the real social difficulties that many people face and to help them to find effective ways of tackling these difficulties.

This initial stage of problem clarification can enable a woman seeking help to begin to construct explicit, clear and realistic models of her problems. However, the experience of being listened to, being taken seriously and being valued by someone is equally important and can, in itself, enhance self-esteem and self-confidence. This will enable the woman to deal more effectively with the problems she is facing.

Setting goals

Based on the understandings reached in stage 1, the changes needed to find reasonable solutions are considered. The helper's role is primarily to encourage the person to devise goals that can be implemented to achieve the desired effects. The aim is to formulate clear, specific goals that are realistic and attainable within a particular period of time. For some problems it is helpful to set a series of goals. A woman might be helped to prioritize and carefully think through the change process and what this would involve. This might include visualizing the effects of change upon her life, and anticipating any difficulties that might arise or act as barriers to success.

To return to the example of Sue, during this stage she focused on how she could help herself. One goal was to question her thoughts about herself as someone who is unattractive and ageing, and rather to think of herself as a young woman who had ovaries that were not working properly. (She had begun to have hormone replacement therapy to reduce the risk or osteoporosis.) This goal was achieved fairly easily. She then began to think more about the future. Her main priority was to make changes in her choice of work. To this end it was agreed, as an initial goal, to continue to meet to discuss options in this area of her life.

In some cases, one might wish to follow through a goal based on a particular model, knowing that there are alternatives. For example, one woman had painful menstrual periods but did not want to take medication if she could avoid it. She decided to try to learn to use relaxation to ease her pain. This goal was based on the model that psychological factors, such as relaxation and distraction, can ameliorate pain experiences.

Making the changes

Having decided upon goals, the next stage deals with how they can best be achieved, putting plans into action and evaluating progress. It can be liberating for people to 'brainstorm' ways of achieving goals, that is, thinking of as many ways as possible and putting forward their own ideas, however silly they might seem. To be supported in this process can enhance a person's confidence. The next step is to look at each option in turn, assessing the relative benefits and costs of each strategy.

Making changes can include planning changes in lifestyle, such as taking more exercise or increasing leisure time, as well as attempting to alter the way a person copes with distress, for example, by discussing problems rather than bottling up feelings. Changes can also include thinking about things from a different perspective, as in Sue's case.

Planning and evaluating various hypothetical actions, as well as the ability to anticipate the outcome of particular options, is essential to good decision-making. The helper's role is to facilitate this process, rather than to provide the answers. The final decision should always rest with the person seeking help.

Once the best available plan is reached, and it may be the case of trying one option first knowing that an alternative is available, the person is given support and encouragement and may also be offered training in specific skills, for example in assertiveness, to achieve the goal.

It is at this stage that there is considerable flexibility in the methods (or counselling approaches) available to the helper to effect change.

Progress is assessed regularly and, if necessary, changes may be made to the plan. Therefore, evaluation is not the last step; it is an ongoing process. It is hoped that the woman seeking help will be able to put her learnt problem-solving skills into practice to maintain achievements and anticipate future problems.

This approach, at its simplest, is a way of looking at problems which can concern emotions or health, or past or future events. The only criteria for helping is that the individual thinks that there is a problem and wishes to be helped. The need for specialist information, and the importance of planning and evaluating treatment choices is also acknowledged. Other models or theoretical approaches can be used within this broad framework. Because of its simplicity, and because many of the problems of women and health care workers in obstetrics and gynaecology concern communication, decision-making and the need for clarification, Egan's model will be used as a broad framework in the chapters that follow.

In the next three chapters communication and counselling skills are discussed further, with practical examples in the area of obstetrics and gynaecology.

Summary

❑ The aims of developing counselling skills are to improve communication, to enable women to be informed and to have personal control over their treatment, to offer support and encouragement, and to help those with particular problems to find solutions and to help themselves.

❑ Communication and counselling skills can be learnt. They include listening, exploring and clarifying problems, setting goals, giving advice and information, as well as support.

❑ The ideal helping relationship is a partnership in which there is mutual participation and respect. Change is facilitated by basic attitudes of respect, genuineness and empathy.

❑ Egan's problem-management approach (a skills-based, eclectic model) is consistent with the biopsychosocial model of the person outlined earlier and is adopted as a general framework in the chapters that follow.

❑ This model has three main stages: 1. The person's understandings and representations of the problem are explored and clarified and alternatives discussed. 2. Based on the implications of the prior discussions, goals are set which are realistic and clearly stated. 3. Changes are planned to achieve the goals, which may be facilitated by a variety of approaches. The outcomes of actions are evaluated and the models modified accordingly.

4

Initial Contact and Exploration

The basic skills of communication and counselling are the focus of this chapter. These include the skills required to establish the helping relationship (for example, attending, listening and demonstrating empathy), as well as those required for the clarification and exploration of problems. Good communication skills can be applied to most situations and, with adequate supervision and training, these skills can be continually improved. The stories of four women, who have been mentioned earlier, are followed in this chapter and in Chapter 6, which is more directly concerned with finding solutions.

The Setting

Before making contact with the person seeking help, it can be useful to take some time to think about the following points which relate to your role and your work setting.

- Do you have access to a private place to talk?
- Will you be free from interruptions?
- Is the room comfortable enough to put the person at ease?
- Are chairs suitably positioned?
- How much time do you have to talk to the person?
- Will you need to perform a physical examination?
- What will the person seeking help be expecting when they see you?

If you are well prepared, you can help to put people at ease and give them a clear idea of what they might expect.

The initial contact with a woman or couple should be carried out, if possible, in a private, congenial and comfortable setting, where there are few or no interruptions. If interruptions do occur, you should apologize and make a determined effort to avoid further distractions. For example, if during the interview the telephone rings and you answer, 'I am sorry, but I'm with someone at the moment. Can I ring you back?', the person is more likely to feel respected than if you continue a long conversation in their presence. Interruptions can usually be avoided by careful planning, such as letting colleagues know that you cannot be contacted until after a certain time.

Privacy is very important; the person should feel comfortable enough to talk without being afraid of being overheard. For example, if you are on a ward, try to use a side room, rather than drawing curtains around a bed. If you use a room, it should have enough space for several chairs and be comfortably lit and heated. Chairs are best positioned at about a 90 degree angle, so that you are facing each other but not directly opposite. A large desk between you can act as a barrier and can reinforce the professional identity of the helper, thereby promoting an expert rather than a helping relationship. The usual distance between people talking is about one or one-and-a-half metres, so this can be used as a guideline for arranging chairs in the room. Use chairs of the same height, in order to reduce any perceived difference in status between the health care worker and the patient.

If a physical examination is part of the initial consultation, talk to the woman while she is sitting down until the presenting problem is clarified. The physical examination can then be carried out in another part of the room. It is important to resume the consultation seated as before, with the patient fully clothed, in order to discuss the problem and its possible treatment further. Women often feel very vulnerable during a vaginal examination and want to know that the doctor/nurse is attending fully to their emotional and physical needs.

If the physical setting is such that there is no possibility for a private conversation, it is far better to explain this and rearrange a meeting at another time, stressing the importance of understanding the person's concerns fully. Time constraints are common in health care settings. Make it clear how much time is available and, if time is limited, make an appointment to take things further on another occasion.

It is obviously important to introduce yourself so that the person understands your position in the hospital or clinic and how you might relate to or differ from other health care workers. Anna works as an abortion counsellor in a teaching hospital. This is an example of how she might introduce herself:

'Good afternoon, Mrs Thomas, pleased to meet you. I am Anna Short. I am a counsellor here and work with the doctor, whom you have already met. I see all women before they arrange to have an abortion and am here to answer any questions you might have and to let you know what it will involve. This should take about 20 to 30 minutes.'

The desired helping relationship (described in Chapter 3) is characterized by an open-ended interviewing style and a person-centred approach. The basic skills required are careful listening, attending and the ability to show empathy.

Attending and Listening

Paying attention to someone is the opposite of ignoring them, and can be comforting in itself. For example, being with someone who is distressed can be helpful even if little is said. Inattention, particularly when a person feels emotionally weak, can be experienced as very painful. Concentrating on the other person can help you to be sensitive to their verbal and non-verbal communications, and the knowledge that they are being heard and given time encourages them to talk.

The helper's non-verbal cues signify to people how much attention they are receiving. It can be useful to be aware of the following in your interactions with patients, colleagues and others.

Posture communicates attention. Sitting at an angle to the person leaning slightly forward in an open way is much better than slouching back in a chair, or sitting with your arms folded tightly in front of you. Try to be relatively relaxed and natural in your behaviour. The posture of the other person will also help to let you know if they are tense or relaxed.

Movements can be distracting and can communicate boredom, impatience or, at worst, rudeness. For example, fiddling with a pen, looking at one's watch, reading through notes or writing are signs of inattention. If you need to look at notes or write something, then it is polite to explain to the person what you are doing and why. Obviously it would be unrealistic to attempt to be completely still, and some movement facilitates conversation. A nod or leaning forward if a person looks distressed, can demonstrate attention. If the person appears restless this should be noted, as they might be holding something back, or be angry or simply concerned about getting home on time. Do not assume that you know what non-verbal behaviour means; it is always best to ask the other person in a non-threatening manner.

Looking at the person is a crucial sign of attention. The person listening should look at the person talking, usually in the direction of their face.

One's gaze should not be fixed, however, and it is quite normal to look away and back again. The direction of looking is determined to a large extent by whether you are talking or listening, and by the material being discussed. The person talking usually looks less directly at the other person, while the listener focuses attention more closely on the speaker. If the topic is anxiety-provoking the speaker is likely to look away more.

Facial expressions reflect mood and emotions. For example, if a person is surprised, angry or tense, it is likely to show, so when attending we constantly monitor the other person's facial expression for cues. Sometimes there is a difference between what a person is saying and his/her facial expression. It may be, for example, that he/she believes that feelings should be controlled, or that some bad news has not yet been internalized. Again you can formulate hypotheses, but never assume that these are true without checking with the person.

Synchrony in conversations signifies attention and interest. This usually develops naturally; that is, people take turns to speak and listen and tend to mirror tone of voice, the amount of eye contact, the speed of speech, pauses and bodily movements.

Attending is also an internal thinking (or cognitive) process. When you are listening other thoughts will sometimes intrude. Attention can be thought of as being aware both of external events (the person and the outside world) and internal events (one's thoughts about the other person and extraneous thoughts). It is clearly important to refocus attention to the person if thoughts wander to different topics or personal concerns.

Listening is a complex and active process which involves making sense of the person's verbal and non-verbal communications. The helper strives to hear what the person is saying and how he/she understands the problems. We do not passively take in a person's story; in any conversation we are constantly looking for underlying meanings and searching for evidence to support our own theories in attempting to understand people around us.

The focus of attention should be primarily upon the woman seeking help and her models of the problem. The aim here is to build up a picture of her internal representations. You will have your own ideas too, but keep these separate in your mind. It helps to try to keep an open mind initially, and to assume that there are a number of possible ways of looking at the problem. You do not have to come up with an answer; your aim is to help the other person to think about her own views.

Given the complexity of this task it is important not to rush; take time to think. Do not move in too quickly with your own theories or focus on the aspect of the problem that you are particularly interested in. This can lead to selective attention, that is, only noticing or hearing those parts of the story that concur with your own ideas. People seeking help are likely to be looking for cues from you about what topics are appropriate to discuss. It can help to prime them by saying, 'I am interested in how you see the problem', so that they feel more confident about telling you what they think is relevant.

Listening means not only hearing what the other person is saying but also noticing their expressions of emotion, tone of voice, and body language. Dawn came to a clinic to have a cervical smear test.

Doctor: *You have had a smear test before haven't you?*

Dawn: *Yes . . . er . . .* (She looked down with her hands held together.)

Doctor: *Is there anything that is worrying you about having this smear test today?*

Dawn: *No, no not really.* (She continued to hold her hands tightly and blushed.)

Doctor: *I notice that you're holding yourself tensely. What are you feeling at the moment?*

Dawn went on to talk about a sexual problem, pain on penetration, which she feared would occur during the examination and which caused her embarrassment. Notice that the doctor in this example did not make an assumption about Dawn's mood, instead she commented on her behaviour or body language, and asked about her feelings. Non-verbal behaviour can sometimes 'leak' messages in situations where the person feels unwilling or unable to say what they really want or feel.

Active listening means involving oneself in what a woman is saying, trying to understand the main message she is giving, what is most important to her, and how she is feeling. You can show that you are listening by using minimal prompts, such as a nod or 'yes', but these can be irritating if they are over-used.

Talking with a woman about her problems may generate all sorts of feelings in you. By trying to identify how you feel, you can sometimes gain understanding about how she might relate to others in her life, for example, family and friends. For instance one woman was very distressed and made it clear that she wanted help. She spoke quickly and described several gynaecological problems, including premenstrual tension, painful periods and concerns about her fertility. The intensity of her feelings, the speed of her speech, and the way she skipped from one problem to another gave neither of us time to think and left me feeling confused. She had seen several doctors and was on the waiting list for surgical treatment. The manner in which she presented her problems may well have confused other health professionals too. We discussed the need to deal with the confusion (which she also acknowledged) and planned to meet to try to clarify the nature of her problems in liaison with her gynaecologist.

There are many barriers or obstacles to good listening. Being distracted by one's own thoughts, feeling tired or ill, being too keen to give advice, talking too much and social or cultural differences, can render listening and understanding difficult. For example, the doctor in Pauline's case (see page 27) felt that his advice was in her best interests, but did not give her time to express her viewpoint. Premature judgement can be offputting. As Pauline said, 'I just put up a barrier'. Listening and understanding do not necessarily mean that you agree with a woman, but show that you are trying to see the situation from her perspective.

Active listening also means making sure that you understand the meanings of words that the person is using. You cannot assume that you share the same meanings, so check that you understand. Communication about patients is often distorted by labels and medical jargon. If someone is described as 'menopausal', 'hysterical' or 'hypochondriacal', the terms act like blinkers and people tend to assume that the label explains all. Such labels are unhelpful and are usually used pejoratively.

As discussed in Chapter 1, it is practically impossible to avoid cultural assumptions and biases in interactions. What you can do though is to try to be aware of your own prejudices and biases. For example, assumptions are continually made about people because of their gender, race, sexual orientation, nationality, social status, religion, politics and/or lifestyle. Question automatic thoughts or judgements! For example, if you have some information about someone that you are going to meet, spend a few minutes imagining them and thinking about your expectations of them on the basis of your knowledge. Then ask yourself why you are making these assumptions and try to approach each person with an open mind. Think about the following examples:

'Ms X is a 50-year-old school teacher . . .'

'Ms Y is a 22-year-old single parent with three children . . .'

'Mrs Z has had three terminations of pregnancies in her twenties, and now at 39 is seeking treatment for infertility . . .'

Peer group discussions can be useful for looking at your beliefs and reactions, for example, to single parenthood, abortion, contraception, and to fertility treatments. Similarly, working with women with reproductive problems requires an examination of one's own thoughts and assumptions about women's roles. It can be easy to feel critical of other people who make different choices, for example, about child care or a career.

Being aware of your own attitudes and feelings, such as envy or disappointment, can help you to avoid acting on such feelings. For example, Debbie, a midwife, was herself undergoing treatment for infertility. She was becoming irritable at work and went home with a headache most nights. Realizing she was under stress, she was encouraged to talk to her nursing officer, who listened and enabled Debbie to express her feelings, her personal disappointments as well as her envy of other women on her ward. She was able to continue with her work and negotiated time off for her own clinic appointments, and, as a result, she felt supported by her nursing officer.

Demonstrating Empathy

Empathy involves both listening and understanding but also communicating one's understanding; showing the other person that you understand how they might be feeling or thinking in the current situation. To be empathic you have to put yourself in the other person's shoes and then convey your thoughts back to them. This can be done by reflecting back, in a simple statement, your understanding of what you think the person is feeling, saying or thinking. A statement, such as, 'So you felt both depressed and angry after you left the clinic', can show that you are listening, and that you are trying to make sense of how the person is feeling. However, you should not be talking too much, but rather listening carefully and commenting occasionally on what is being said.

Demonstrating empathy in this way does not mean that you will be accurate all the time, and an important function of empathic statements is to check that your understandings are roughly on the right lines. Moreover, because your perceptions are likely to be inaccurate some of the time, it is important that your statements are made tentatively (for example, 'It looks as though . . .'; 'It sounds as if . . .' or 'So you're saying that . . .'), so that the woman feels able to correct you or elaborate her position.

Empathic statements are not questions, although they usually elicit a response. The resulting communication becomes a joint task of achieving a shared understanding of the thoughts and feelings of the woman seeking help; and this process itself can increase her sense of self-worth.

There is an important difference between empathy and sympathy. Sympathy has more in common with pity or compassion and implies some agreement with the other's point of view. Empathy is an attempt to understand how the person feels or thinks and opens the discussion to looking at problems further. Sympathy, on the other hand, can serve to maintain the status quo, and may leave the person feeling patronized. You may feel compelled to rush in and offer advice and sympathy, but it is usually more helpful to listen and let the person talk.

Do not try to overinterpret what you think might be the causes of the person's feelings or behaviour. It is always better to stay with the more obvious messages that they are giving you. For example, Maggie is at home with a three-year-old daughter and ten-day-old son. When her health visitor (HV) arrives, the baby is unsettled and her daughter is wanting to play.

Maggie: *The baby's fine you know, but there's a lot to do. He doesn't sleep very regularly, and when he is asleep, Beth* (her daughter) *wants me all to herself.* (Picks up baby, HV plays with Beth.)

HV: *And how have you been feeling yourself?* (Open question.)

Maggie (laughs): *Exhausted.* (Pause.) *No really, it's harder this time round. It's not just physically, it's emotionally draining too. I feel as if I'm trying to please everyone and not getting it right. Sometimes I just have to walk out of the room to escape from all their demands.*

HV: *It seems to all get a bit overwhelming at times.* (Demonstrates empathy.)

Maggie: *Yes.*

They went on to discuss play groups for Beth and ways for Maggie and her husband to share time with the children at weekends and in the evenings.

Pauline (see page 27) talked to me after her hysterectomy. She recalled her conversation with her doctor before the operation.

Pauline: *When he said that, I just put up a barrier. He made me feel like a silly little girl. I still feel angry about it.*

MH: *Yes I can see that you are.* (Demonstrating empathy.)

Jen lost her baby seven months ago (see page 47) and began to talk about her thoughts and feelings to her doctor (D).

Jen: *I don't really talk about him much at all. At the beginning Dave* (her husband) *and I looked at the photo together at home but I'd just cry . . . and now over time we've both stopped doing that. I suppose we're avoiding it.* (Looks tearful and about to cry.)

D: *But the feelings are still very much with you.* (Demonstrating empathy.)

Jen (cries): *Yes . . . You see I daren't let myself cry because I don't want to upset Dave or embarrass myself at work . . . you know.*

She is given time to cry and recover in the session.

Demonstrating empathy will not take away distress or solve problems, but it encourages women seeking help to explore these issues and builds up the helping relationship. Empathic responses also help to clarify core messages or problems. For example, Pauline talked about her angry feelings regarding her doctor's remarks and, in an earlier conversation, expressed anger and distress about having to have a hysterectomy at all.

MH: *So you seem to be feeling angry partly with Dr N for his way of talking with you, and also about having to have the operation.*

Pauline (long pause): *Separating the issues, anger with him as a person and feelings about the operation and fertility, does make it a bit easier to deal with.*

So far I have recommended that you try to:
• listen carefully
• give yourself time to think
• try to put yourself in the position of the woman seeking help
• demonstrate empathy
• remember that you are there to help her to look at her problems
• monitor your own feelings, attitudes and biases.

Try not to:
• be judgemental
• talk too much
• overinterpret
• rush in to offer advice or sympathy
• be distracted by personal problems or act on personal biases.

These skills can be practised with friends and colleagues using role-play or video-taped feedback, taking turns acting the roles of patient and helper. Staff training, if carried out in a relaxed and supportive setting with constructive feedback, is crucial to the development and maintenance of counselling skills. (See Chapter 7 for discussion of training and supervision.)

Problem Clarification

Here the aim is to help the woman to tell her story. Try to use open questions that enable you to explore her feelings, experience or behaviour. Examples of open questions include:

- 'How are you feeling?'
- 'What did you do at that time?'
- 'How did you deal with that?'
- 'What are you expecting now?'
- 'What thoughts do you have about that?'

A nurse goes to see Mrs Hill on a gynaecology ward. Mrs Hill is going to have a laparoscopy to investigate why she is not conceiving. She has already had a series of unsuccessful hormonal treatments.

Nurse: *Good afternoon, Mrs Hill. I am Jenny and I will be taking care of you today. You are having a laparoscopy tomorrow morning. How are you feeling about that?*

Mrs Hill: *A bit nervous actually. The doctor told me a bit about it. I'm not so bothered about the operation, it's the results that worry me. When will I find out?*

Nurse: *The consultant will come to see you probably tomorrow evening and tell you what they have found. Is there anything else that you are unsure about?*

Some people talk freely, but others, especially if they feel embarrassed, anxious or vulnerable, may be more reticent. There are several ways of encouraging people to talk, but this does not mean that you should always try to fill silences. Pauses are often useful times to think. You can help a woman to explore her problems by:

Asking open questions:
'You mentioned that you were worried about going into labour. Can you tell me a bit more about your concerns?'

Asking for clarification:
'What does it mean for you when you say you've been feeling low?'

'Premenstrual tension can mean different things to different people. Can you tell me what happens for you?'

'I can see that you're anxious about the examination, but I'm not sure why.'

Asking for an example:
'You said that at times you feel unable to cope with the baby. Can you give me an example and tell me what actually happens?'

Reflecting back or echoing:
Jen: *When I think about him* (her stillborn baby) *I feel as if I'm going to explode inside.*

Helper: *Explode inside?*

Jen: *Well yes, really. The feeling is so strong I actually worry that something terrible will happen.*

These ways of responding and encouraging help you to follow the person's story. It is important to avoid certain types of questions, particularly those which are leading or value-laden. For example:

'Do you think you're depressed because you've reached the menopause?' (Leading question.)

'Do you feel guilty about having the abortion?' (Value-laden question.)

These questions contain assumptions which put the woman in a difficult position. By answering the question she is forced to take your position on board. Similarly, it can be disturbing if personal, intimate or sexual questions are asked too soon, in a confrontational manner or without adequate explanation. Hilary went to see her gynaecologist because intercourse was painful. The doctor (D), noticed that she was tense and spent some time trying to clarify the problem, as well as helping her to be calmer:

D: *How can I help you?* (Open question.)

Hilary: *Well, it's been going on for almost a year now, since I had Dawn* (her baby) *. . . You know when we try to make love . . . well it just doesn't work out.* (Looks sad.)

D: *And this has been getting you down.* (Demonstrates empathy.)

Hilary: *Yes I've felt much worse recently. Well, she's one now; I should be OK. I mean it was fine before.*

D: *So before Dawn was born there were no problems and you enjoyed lovemaking.* (Reflecting back.)

Hilary: *We'd make love about twice a week. I enjoyed it and Ron said he did. I did get a bit tense sometimes though and that made it hard for him . . . you know to . . . um . . .*

D: *To penetrate.*

Hilary: *Yes, and really that's the problem now.*

This doctor took time to put Hilary at ease before encouraging her to talk about the sexual problem. If he had said, 'Well, tell me first exactly what the problem is', there may have been less rapport. He helped her by offering the term 'penetrate' when she was uncertain about what would be appropriate. However, if semi-medical terms, such as coitus, vaginismus, clitoris, premature ejaculation, impotence, are used, it is vital to explain in your own words what these words mean. Diagrams can be a useful aid. A rule of thumb is to use the same words as the woman if you feel comfortable with this but make sure that you make clear what you mean. Clarifying terms in this way can also reduce feelings of embarrassment and awkwardness.

It is important to follow the patient's lead when clarifying the nature of the problem. Do this by listening, checking that you understand by using empathic statements, and summarizing the main issues that have been raised.

Summarizing can be a useful way of rounding off an interview and serves to provide an overview of what has been said, and a shared understanding of the problem. Summaries should be clear and brief, bringing ideas and thoughts together. Feeding back the person's view in this way can encourage them to question the accuracy of their assumptions and theories. For example, a health visitor offered the following summary to a woman who was exhausted a week after giving birth.

'Am I right in thinking, then, that you are feeling exhausted and this is making it hard for you to get through the day? This might be caused by several factors. First, the labour was very long and the baby was overdue. Second, for various reasons you have had less support than you expected. Third, you had expected the baby to sleep all the time and to feed without any problems. Does that sound right to you?'.

A summary presents an outline of the person's model of the problem, as you understand it so far, and should include the following:

- The nature of the problem.
- The impact of the problem.
- The main factors causing or influencing the problem.

In this way a shared, initial understanding is reached, which can be challenged and modified later if appropriate. Challenging skills and exploration of alternative models are discussed in Chapter 6.

Depending upon the context, clarifying the main concerns and checking back that you understand may be all that is needed. For example, on a maternity ward, listening to an expectant mother's feelings and expectations about labour, and then explaining the procedures and what help can be expected, can in itself be highly beneficial. Undue anxiety can be noted, and steps taken to give extra support during labour. As illustrated repeatedly in Chapter 2, women appreciate and remember staff who in their daily work show understanding and respect.

Before going on to explore the problem further, it is necessary to establish whether this is appropriate and whether a woman wishes to do so. Exploration of her expectations, the particular context, as well as being honest about your own level of expertise, are useful guides. There are no hard and fast rules, but at some point in the initial contact, usually after the woman has described her main problems, some kind of contract is negotiated. This would include an agreement about whether any further meetings are necessary and the purpose of these. At this stage the notion of a partnership can be discussed. The initial agreement can be temporary, to be renegotiated at a later date. For example, you may not have had adequate time to understand the nature of the problem, so you might arrange to meet again for a further discussion. It is important to resist the urge to offer help or treatment before properly understanding the problem.

Ending an initial contact is made easier if you are clear at the beginning how much time you have. This will vary depending on the setting. Let the person know how long you have left five or ten minutes before you have to stop, so that there is time for you to summarize and to agree what to do next. If someone has been upset during the discussion, warning of the end of the meeting can give them some time to compose themselves.

Further Exploration

Depending upon the situation and the nature of the problem, further exploration may take place during an initial contact and subsequent meetings.

People seeking help come with certain expectations and beliefs. Their personalities, coping skills and their social context will determine the type of help they feel best able to use. Some may have unrealistic hopes, because they believe that medicine can cure all ills, while others may feel resentful or critical of people, such as doctors, who hold positions of authority. Enquiry about such expectations and theories of the causes of the problem, using open questions, can help to understand how a woman is making sense of her situation.

Asking open questions enables you to pursue the issues the patient considers important. However, it is also helpful to have a framework of areas tht you might want to explore, not necessarily in any fixed order, as a guide. The following questions are based on the areas outlined in the biopsychosocial model (see page 9).

- How does she describe the nature of the problem?
- When did it begin?
- What was happening in her life at the time it began?
- What did she think was causing it at that time?
- How frequently does it occur now?
- Does it occur, or become worse, in particular situations?
- What does she think and feel when it occurs?
- How does the problem affect her life in general, for example, relationships, self-esteem, work?
- What, in her view, are the main causes of or influences on this problem now?
- What has she found helpful or unhelpful?
- How does she deal with the problem?
- Are there any other problems or stresses in her life?
- When she went to see her doctor what did she expect?
- How much control, if any, does she feel she has over the problem?

There are ways of enabling people to talk about their thoughts and lives, some of which have already been discussed. Remember the following guidelines:

- Follow where the woman leads.
- Prime her to think in terms of models or theories.
- Explain why you are asking certain things.
- Try to link an area that you wish to explore with what has been previously discussed.
- Ask for clarification and check that your understandings are correct.
- Be tentative and encourage the woman to express her own thoughts.

Priming the person to elaborate theories means making explicit the assumption that there may be different ways of understanding problems, and different possible causal explanations. For example,

'There are several possible reasons for irregular periods. What do you think might be happening?'. Some people find it easier to begin by describing how they understood the problem when it first began. You might then enquire as to whether this explanation has changed over time and in what way.

Asking questions about people's personal lives, such as relationships or past histories, can be threatening and can appear inappropriate. It is important, therefore, to explain why you want to enquire about certain areas, and to make links, if possible, with the previous conversation. For example, if a woman has been describing her severe hot flushes, you can say, 'Sometimes people feel that their flushes get worse when they feel stressed; I was wondering if this happens for you'. This may lead to a discussion of her lifestyle. If you are aware of a past event such as childhood sexual abuse or rape wait until the woman is ready to talk about it, rather than introduce the topic yourself. Also don't assume that one past event is necessarily the sole cause of a woman's current problems.

Women seeking fertility treatments or abortions might well feel distressed or angry if asked detailed questions about previous relationships without adequate explanation, or without permission being asked. For example, Carol interpreted her doctor's question about her past as inferring that she was psychologically abnormal. 'He asked me about my relationship with my mother. I said it wasn't too good but whose is and anyway I had gone to see him because of the PMT. It felt intrusive as if he was criticizing me'. Similarly, Joan was taken aback by her doctor's comments when she was having an internal examination. 'He touched my stomach in a way that made me flinch. It tickled really. Then straight away he asked me if I'd had any traumatic experiences in the past'. In this case the doctor failed to enquire from Joan how she felt and why she might have reacted as she did before asking a loaded question.

Case Studies

The stories of four women are included here to illustrate further explorations of problems. Carol, 26, presented PMT as her main problem (see page 35); Janet, 24, described how her pelvic pain had worsened since the death of her friend (see page 18); Jen, 28, was having difficulties containing her distress following the loss of her baby seven months before (see page 47); and Pauline, 37, experienced depression and anger following major surgery, which included hysterectomy (see page 27).

Carol

Carol had described her experience of PMT as 'feeling drained, tense and depressed about my life in general'. Initially when she spoke to Sister J. (SJ) she had described this as the main problem and had wanted medical treatment. The interview continued:

SJ: *So before your period you feel bad about your life in general. Can you say a bit more about this and how you feel when you feel bad?*

Carol: *Well, I feel as if I haven't achieved much. I get anxious about going out and don't mix much.* (Looks down.)

SJ: *It looks as if you feel sad about it at the moment.*

Carol: *Well I do when I really think about it. Most of the time I keep busy at home. I just try to keep going day to day.*

SJ: *So most of the time you try not to think.* (Pause.) *How do you cope with the feelings when you can't avoid them?*

Carol: *That's what happens before my period. It's harder to cope.* (Pause.) *Then, . . . well I drink and smoke cigarettes . . . I suppose that doesn't help too much either.*

At this point Carol had shifted slightly away from describing her problems entirely in terms of PMT, her initial theory, and began to see herself as someone who perhaps had more general problems in her life, which she found harder to cope with before her period. Following her lead, showing empathy and asking for clarification enabled the conversation to flow fairly naturally. She went on to look at her ways of dealing with her distress (avoidance, alcohol and cigarettes), acknowledging that these were coping strategies unlikely to lead to positive change.

Janet

Janet, 24, was referred to me by her gynaecologist to see if I could help her manage her pain, a problem which she had had for four years and which was increasingly affecting her life. She had undergone several investigations which revealed no clear organic cause. I had been introduced to her before and had scheduled the session that follows:

MH: *I know that you have seen a lot of different people. I wondered how you must be feeling about coming to see me here today.* (Exploring expectations.)

Janet: *Well really I'm not sure why I'm here. The doctor said you might be able to help me . . . but no-one else has so far.* (Pause.)

MH: *You feel a bit disillusioned with doctors and hospitals.* (Demonstrating empathy.)

Janet: *I do really . . . no-one's found a cause of my pain . . . There must be something wrong . . . and then he* (the doctor) *said to see you . . . being a psychologist. To me that was him saying you're imagining it.* (Looks upset.)

MH: *It is important that you told me that, because I want to stress that in my view all pain is real. I do believe that you have pain.* ·

I go on to explain that new thinking and research about pain shows that it is influenced by many factors and discuss the Gate Control Theory (see page 40) with her, giving examples of how pain is influenced by attention and mood and how reactions to pain can feed back to open the gate to pain impulses.

It could be argued that it would have been better to explore Janet's own theories about the cause of her pain before presenting a multi-dimensional pain model. However, I felt that it was important to clarify my position *vis-à-vis* her pain, in order to put her at ease and establish a working relationship. Later in the interview we discussed her theories and the psychosocial context.

MH: *Your ideas may have changed over time, but what do you yourself think might be giving you pain?*

Janet: *I've always had painful periods but lately I've been getting pains in the middle of the month as well. I suppose I've thought it must be something to do with my hormones but it has got worse . . . gradually.*

MH: *Gradually . . .*

Janet: *Well I could cope with it until about six months ago.*

MH: *And what was happening in your life then?*

Janet: *Nothing, really . . .* (Pause.) *There was an accident . . .*

She continued to talk about the road traffic accident in which her friend had been killed. Janet was the passenger.

Janet: *If only I had told her to slow down . . . I've been so bad since, the pain is so much worse . . .* (Becomes tearful.)

MH: *I can see that it is still very difficult to talk about.* (Demonstrating empathy.)

Janet: *I haven't really talked about it since it happened. Her parents cut me off . . . and my family's attitude is to not talk about things like that.*

Janet went on to describe her current situation and her family life. She described feeling tension in her abdomen, and the difficulty she had sleeping. She lives at home with her parents. Her older sister is married with a child. She said she found it difficult to talk to her family about her feelings and particularly about the accident. She recalled that her mother was attentive when she was in pain, but this was mainly by doing things for her, for example, making her hot drinks and giving her painkillers, rather than listening.

Our shared understanding of her problems, at this point, was that although the initial cause of the pain was unclear, it had become much worse following a stressful life event (the accident). In addition, the way her distress was being communicated at home, and the family's reaction to her pain, might well be making her feel more distressed and unsupported.

This example illustrates how important it is to find out about the person's expectations. Janet's concerns were that I had a rigid psychological view of her problems, so it was necessary to discuss a more complex model early in the interview.

Jen

Jen decided that she needed help, and went to talk to her doctor (D), when she found that her feelings of grief about the loss of her baby (see pages 47 and 68) were becoming difficult to control. She described how she avoided situations that might trigger her grief, and how she did not discuss the baby in order to protect her husband.

D: *Can you say a bit more about how dealing with your feelings in this way is affecting your daily life?*

Jen: *I go to fewer family gatherings . . . my brother's got young children. I just find it difficult.*

D: *Difficult . . .*

Jen: *I feel as if they are very aware of me and yet no-one says anything. The atmosphere is tense and really I'm on edge in case anything sets me off.*

D (pauses): *You're afraid of losing control.*

Jen: *That's right. The feelings are so strong I think I'll explode or something, or that no-one will be able to deal with me.*

D: *So are you saying that one of the fears about talking is that no-one can deal with it. But it's difficult to let yourself find out about that at the moment.*

Jen (pauses): *I know deep down that I'm not helping myself by trying to push it all away.*

In the rest of the session she described the circumstances surrounding the loss of her baby, whom she and her husband, Dave, had named Thomas. Jen began labour unexpectedly while Dave was at a conference. Thomas died during labour; Jen held the baby afterwards and they arranged a funeral for him.

Jen: *After we left the hospital I still felt numb. Dave did everything for me. Then I got the flu quite badly . . . I was a bit delirious, I think, for a couple of weeks. It was then that everyone came to see me and I wasn't really there. After that Dave changed jobs and I felt as if I had to be strong for him. We just put on brave faces I suppose, but it hasn't got any easier.*

The circumstances following the loss of her baby had, in a way, served to maintain her avoidance of painful feelings. Her doctor went on to explore Jen's feelings of grief.

D: *Did you have any ideas or expectations about how you might feel in the months that followed?*

Jen: *I've never lost anyone before. I knew that really I'd never get over it and I suppose feeling that, I didn't try to bring the feelings out . . .* (Pause.) *In a strange way keeping him all locked inside me has let me hold on to him . . .* (Looks tearful.) *No-one told me how strong the feelings would be, or how isolated I'd feel . . .* (Cries and then gradually stops.)

D: *I can see it is very difficult indeed, but I'm pleased you have been able to talk as you have and you're still in one piece.* (Reference to her fear of exploding.)

Jen: *Yes . . .* (Laughs.)

In this interview Jen described how her problems were affecting her life and how she was coping with her distress by trying to control her feelings and by avoiding situations which might precipitate them. It seemed important that the difficulties she was having in talking in the interview were acknowledged, and that it was pointed out how her fears were not borne out when she did discuss her feelings in this setting. There were quite a few pauses which were useful for both Jen and her doctor to think, and for Jen to deal with her distress.

Pauline

I had talked to Pauline on two occasions after her hysterectomy during which she expressed strong mixed feelings both about having to have the operation, and about the way in which her doctor had treated her. She felt belittled by him and had been relatively unprepared before the operation. After a long talk with her doctor, during which she put over her point of view, she had been able to separate her anger with him from the impact of the operation. In what follows, we explored the impact of the operation upon her relationships and lifestyle, as well as her ways of coping with distress. Pauline had been telling me about her discussions with her doctor, but still felt very upset. I wanted to understand more about what was upsetting her and how she was currently viewing what had happened.

MH: *When you're feeling like this what kind of thoughts go through your mind?*

Pauline: *It's more the infertility now; having no chance of a baby. It's affecting my feelings towards Ben* (her boyfriend). *I feel like pushing him away. I am irritable with him.* (Pause.) *He tells me he doesn't mind but I don't believe him. In a couple of years he might change his mind . . . and will want someone else.*

MH (pauses): *Are you saying that you're concerned that he might reject you in the future, and that that fear makes you distant from him now?*

Pauline: *Maybe . . . I've always been in control and independent. I suppose being like this is hard for me.*

MH: *In what ways is it hard for you?*

Pauline: *Usually I'm in charge and act strong, you know. I'm in a very responsible position at work and after my divorce I had to cope with all the finances and everything. Being in hospital and being ill is just hard for me . . .*

MH: *Do you mean being ill in hospital makes you see that you have weakness, like everyone else, but most of the time you see yourself as having to be very strong.*

Pauline: *Yes . . . I do . . . sort of know that it's a bit of an act. I am strong, but I've always really felt unloved deep down.* (Looks upset.)

MH: *Yes.* (Sits forward.) *Do you want to talk more about that now . . .?*

In this interview I repeated what I thought Pauline was meaning in my my own words, to try to make sure that I understood. It was also necessary to clarify statements like 'being like this is hard for me', because I was unsure about what this meant. When she began to talk about feeling unloved and became upset, I gave her the choice as to whether she wanted to proceed to talk about her past, especially as she had just said that she prefers to be in control.

In fact, she continued to describe how her parents had moved to England from Jamaica after she was born, leaving her in Jamaica to be brought up by a friend of the family. She remembered being badly treated. Her brothers and sisters were looked after by grandparents. After being reunited with her parents when she was 12 her mother gave her lots of attention and she became the favourite; she strived hard at school and became the family success. However, she had not talked about how difficult it had been for her.

Her current distress appeared to have several possible causes. She agreed that her reactions to the operation were influenced by poor communication, as well as the impact of the surgery upon her fertility, and her current relationship. In addition, the experience of being in hospital had made her feel vulnerable, rather than the strong person she usually attempted to be, and she had remembered sad events of the past.

Pauline's, Jen's, Carol's and Janet's stories are continued in Chapter 6, which deals with goal-setting and making changes (Egan's stages 2 and 3).

But discussions with people seeking help do not always run smoothly. The final part of this chapter is concerned with ways of dealing with distress and anger.

Dealing with Distress

The situations and problems that lead to distress are many and varied. It may be worth considering the following as general guidelines when someone is distressed.

- Find a private place to talk.
- Give the person time to cry.
- Empathize and offer support.
- Give the person your full attention.
- Resist the urge to act or to give advice.
- Let the person talk in their own time and follow the person's lead.
- Gradually explore how they are feeling and the reasons for their distress.
- Give the person time and, if necessary, a place to recover, and discuss what happens next.

It is natural to try to relieve someone's distress by holding back information or trying to do something about it quickly. However, these reactions are not always very helpful. In a crisis some health workers rush around sending for other professional staff and arranging for procedures to take place. For example, in the case of detected fetal abnormality, staff can sometimes rush in very quickly to arrange an abortion (partly to relieve their own feelings of impotence or failure). Similarly, a common response to someone who has miscarried is, 'Oh well never mind you can try for another'. This is reassuring for the person saying it, but this type of comment often invalidates a woman's feelings of sadness and regret.

It is not helpful to see outcomes such as pregnancy loss as a personal failure. Rather aim to deal well with difficult situations. In these contexts the woman will experience many strong feelings. In most cases you can help simply by being there. Listening, offering some support and empathy are invaluable qualities at such times and are very much appreciated. People often need permission to cry, to feel that it is acceptable. Women who have experienced loss often say that they found it particularly helpful when staff members showed some of their own feelings. Pat lost her baby shortly after birth:

'It made the whole thing more real for me when she was upset. She put her arm on mine and it helped me to see that my own reactions were normal.'

If someone becomes acutely distressed on a ward or when you are talking with them, the best you can do is to acknowledge, respect and permit them to express their emotions, for example: 'This is really hard, isn't it. Come and sit down here with me'.

Find a private, quiet place to talk where you can gently enquire about the problem, for example: 'Do you feel able to talk about it?' It is important to continue to ask open questions to elicit further anxieties or causes of distress. You do not always have to give advice or information in these situations; in many instances all you should do is be there and listen. This, in itself, is extremely valuable.

Joan, a student nurse, finds Maria crying in a side room on the maternity ward. Maria's baby is asleep on her knee.

Joan: *Maria, I was wondering where you were. How are you today?*

Maria (rubs eyes quickly and smiles): *Oh, I'm fine. I was just resting.* (Gets up and makes her way to the door.)

Joan: *Good, well I'll see you later.*

In this interaction Joan does not acknowledge Maria's tears and Maria does not attempt to discuss the problem. An alternative scenario could be:

Joan: *Maria, I was wondering where you were.* (Sits down.) *You're not feeling too good, I see.*

Maria (smiles): *No not really.* (Tears well up in her eyes.)

Joan: *What is it?*

Maria: *I don't know. He seems fine* (the baby). *I just feel so sad.* (Pause.) (Joan leans forward and strokes the baby.)

Joan: *Do you have any worries about him?*

Maria: *Feeding is a bit difficult . . . he sometimes has a reasonable amount but sometimes he doesn't seem to want any.*

Joan: *Well that sounds fairly normal really . . . Is there anything else?*

Maria: *My family . . . My husband has to work long shifts at the moment and my parents were to come from Greece . . . He* (her husband) *phoned last night and told me they couldn't come now. My father is ill.* (Cries.) *I wanted them to see him – their first grandchild.*

Joan (pauses): *I bet they're feeling bad about it too.*

Here Joan showed empathy and gave Maria time to feel able to talk about her problem. Although Joan couldn't provide a solution, listening helped Maria to put her disappointment into perspective and not feel rejected by her parents.

As described in the previous section, it is important to end meetings properly, giving adequate notice, summarizing, and discussing what happens next. If you are working on a ward or in an out-patient clinic, a follow-up appointment or visit should be offered. Having begun to develop a relationship of trust, it is obviously best if the same health care worker is able to meet the person again, at the very least to enquire how they are as an expression of support and concern.

Dealing with Anger

When you are used to being in a caring or helping role, it can be very difficult when someone you are trying to help, or a relative, becomes angry. Again, there are no simple answers, but the following points are worth considering:

- Listen to what the person has to say.
- Acknowledge their anger.
- Give time for feelings to be expressed.

- Respond by trying to understand what has happened to make them angry, rather than becoming defensive and angry yourself.
- Be honest and apologize if you have made a mistake, and do what you can to prevent this happening again.
- If the person's anger is in reaction to a loss or a diagnosis, try not to take this personally.
- End the interview with a summary of what you both see as the main reasons for the anger and a definite plan of what happens next, be it a follow-up appointment or a change in the treatment plan.
- Afterwards, take time to relax and think about how you coped with the situation; you can do this alone or with a colleague.

No matter how rejected or inadequate you feel, you should try not to respond with anger or by being defensive. Instead acknowledge the other person's anger, empathize and take it seriously, before trying to understand the possible reasons.

Lynda's gynaecologist asked her to see me because she was depressed. She had already been for hormone treatment because she and her GP wondered whether her problems were to do with the menopause.

Lynda: *I have to say I've no idea why she asked me to see you. It's ridiculous. I went for hormone treatment and here I am seeing a psychiatrist or whatever. I'm not going mad you know . . .*

MH: *I can see you feel misunderstood and angry about that.*

Lynda: *I do . . . Well! What can you do for me then?*

MH: *I'm not sure yet . . . perhaps we can start, at least, by trying to look at how this misunderstanding happened.*

Lynda proceeded to talk about the reasons she had gone to her GP and her theories about her complaints, which were hot flushes, having little energy and feeling tired.

Anne and her husband (Carlton) saw her doctor for her six week check after having her baby. She was angry about her treatment in hospital. Two scenarios are described. In the first the doctor (D) behaves defensively:

Carlton: *I want to start by telling you that we have several serious complaints to make about Anne's care — or lack of it — in your ward. Really it's scandalous. The right hand obviously didn't know what the left hand was doing.*

D: *We all do our best here. You would be lucky to find better care in any other district general hospital.*

Carlton: *That's not the point. Your best obviously isn't good enough.* (Gets very angry.) *My wife asked for her waters not to be broken – they were. On three occasions staff made unnecessary, uncaring remarks to her when she was upset and she received contradictory advice about feeding.* (Standing up.)

D: *Wait a minute . . . the baby's fine isn't he . . . ?*

Couple walk to the door.

In an alternative scenario, the doctor acknowledges the anger and attempts to explore the reasons for it.

D: *I am sorry that you feel so distressed by your experience at the hospital. Please do go on and tell me why.*

Carlton: *Well, first of all in my wife's birth plan she asked for her waters not to be broken . . .*

The conversation went on to cover the reasons why the couple were dissatisfied. The doctor listened and arranged to take steps to investigate the problem raised. They agreed on a follow up time to receive the feedback from the investigations.

It is important to give people time to voice their concerns. If you concentrate on listening and trying to understand their anger, you will probably be less likely to react defensively. Try to be as objective as possible. For example, if the person criticizes a colleague or another hospital, try to understand how the person views the situation and reflect this back, rather than agreeing before you have explored other possible explanations for what went wrong. However, it is equally important to admit to mistakes and apologize for them. One way of showing that you take the feedback seriously is to discuss what steps you can take to avoid repetition of the event. For example, a couple attending an infertility clinic were angry because they had had to wait much longer than they had expected. The discussion ended as follows: 'So it seems that the situation could have been partly avoided on that occasion if we started the clinic on time. I will do all I can to prevent this happening again. If we are running late, I will let people in the waiting room know, so that they can go out and come back if they choose'.

Anger is a common reaction to frustration and loss and bad news. It is quite normal to feel angry and upset at the same time in these situations. However, frequently there is no obvious person to blame, for example, for a miscarriage or an unsuccessful fertility treatment. Acknowledging this difficulty and the fact that these feelings are normal, can help. There may be more than one reason why someone is angry. For example, not seeing the doctor you expected because she/he is ill, can feel like the last straw if you have spent all afternoon waiting for trains and buses, having had difficulty making arrangements for childcare and taking leave from work. So, it is worth exploring all possible reasons for the anger.

If you feel that you are becoming angry yourself, there are a few things that you can do. Take a deep breath and try to relax. Don't rush in and argue back; instead, remember that you are there to make sense of the situation, whether you are at fault or not. Make statements to try to clarify why the person feels so strongly. If at the end of the meeting you still have not reached a shared view of what happened, make it clear that you will give what has been said serious thought, and that you would like to arrange another time for further discussion.

The Need to Practise

The tasks and skills discussed in this chapter require practice, and ideally, peer supervision and feedback. When mastered they can be used to facilitate communication with colleagues, as well as people seeking help. Health care workers and others in helping roles themselves often need support in order to find adaptive ways of dealing with stress (see Burnard, 1991). In many situations there are no easy answers to people's problems, and staff at all levels can benefit from sharing their experiences and practising communication skills. Training, supervision and support are discussed more fully in Chapter 7.

Summary

❑ The initial contact should be planned with consideration given to the setting. Ensure privacy and adequate time, which should be free from interruptions and distractions.

❑ The desired helping relationship is characterized by the fundamental attitudes of genuineness, respect and empathy.

❑ These attitudes encourage a sense of self-worth and self-efficacy in the woman seeking help (that is, a confidence in her own ability to make changes).

❑ These fundamental attitudes can be communicated by attending, listening and demonstrating empathy. These are the basic skills or building blocks of counselling and communication because they help to establish a good relationship with the person, and begin the process of exploration of problems.

❑ Exploration of problems means posing open questions, asking for clarification and for examples, reflecting back and summarizing. Follow the person's lead and check back your understandings.

❑ Try to avoid asking leading questions and be aware of your own prejudices and biases.

❑ Offer the woman the opportunity to discuss her expectations, beliefs and theories about her problems. It can help to prime her to think in terms of models, and to explain why you are asking particular questions.

❑ During the initial contact a contract is negotiated so that there is an agreement about what is to be discussed at the time, or what happens next; for example, whether to meet again and the purpose of the meetings.

❑ The ending of the interview should be anticipated, so that you can let the person know when they have a few minutes left. This can give time for a summary, or for any final questions, as well as time to recover if distressing topics have been discussed.

❑ Ways of understanding and dealing with people's distress and anger are described. It is important to listen, give the person time, concentrate on trying to understand how they feel (empathize) and why they feel as they do (exploration). Be honest if you have made a mistake but try not to become defensive and do not feel that you necessarily have to *do* something.

5

Providing Information
and Support

Having considered the communication skills required to understand reproductive problems, this chapter deals specifically with the steps that can be taken to help women to be informed about their problems and treatments. In Chapter 2 women repeatedly expressed the desire for information and full explanations. This was particularly the case when they were anticipating investigations and surgical interventions, procedures which are common in this area of health care. Knowledge is necessary to acquire reasonably accurate expectations, to challenge inaccurate beliefs, to make informed decisions and to prepare psychologically for the future, be it for surgery, labour or dealing with a chronic condition. The need for support was also voiced, especially when receiving bad news, when interventions were stressful, or when it was unavailable from other sources. Indeed, the provision of information and support should go hand in hand, if, as is advocated here, the counselling skills described in previous chapters underpin all meetings between health care workers and people seeking help.

Providing information is one way in which a person's model or understanding of their problems is altered. In acute situations, for example receiving bad news, women and couples are often forced to alter their expectations and their views of the world quite rapidly. Good communication and support are essential in these settings. This chapter deals, in general, with helping people to deal with acute situations, such as diagnostic interventions, gynaecological surgery, childbirth and pregnancy loss. The next chapter deals with helping people to consider alternative models and problem-solving when dealing with more persistent issues.

Guidelines for Providing Information

Opinion surveys over the past 20 years show that a considerable proportion of patients are dissatisfied with the information they are given in health care settings. With the rapid turnover in in-patient wards, many are not adequately informed about their treatment and how to cope during recovery, and many are not aware that they have choices about treatments or procedures. Ill-health, anxiety and fatigue can contribute to an inability to process what information is given. Even when clinicians attempt to give adequate information, a proportion of patients remain dissatisfied. This is likely to be to do with the way in which the information is given, as well as diffidence about asking questions in clinical settings, where people often feel more vulnerable and dependent.

Information is vital if people are to have more independence and control over their health. However, it is important to consider the type of information needed, and how, when and in what form it is best provided. The following are general guidelines about providing information:

- Start by finding out what the person already knows. Explore their view of the problem, their expectations, their fears and their current knowledge.
- Try to be clear and comprehensible. Avoid using jargon or complex medical terminology. Explain terms.
- Do not give too much information. It should be simple, concise and to the point. The greater the number of statements given, the smaller the percentage of information recalled. Information given first and statements which are seen as important are remembered best.
- Group pieces of information together in categories, such as condition, treatment, prognosis, how to cope.
- It is often helpful to give information in more than one form, for example, it might be given in written leaflets or diagrams, as well as verbally.
- Let the person know that you are there to answer their questions.
- Arrange for relatives to help those with learning difficulties and interpreters for those who do not speak the language used.
- Do not make assumptions about who will want or benefit from information based upon social class, age, sexual orientation or ethnic group.
- Repeat the information given and find out whether it has been understood. Ask the person what they understand, how they feel about the information and whether there is anything that they are unclear about.

Giving Bad News

Giving bad news is never easy. Having to tell someone that they have cancer, that their baby has died, or that they cannot have children, is inevitably difficult for all concerned. The aim here is to try to handle these situations with sensitivity and warmth, and to offer clear information, with enough time for tears and further questions.

Sheila describes how her doctor told her that she had cancer. She went to a hospital for examination having had a cervical smear test.

'I wasn't worried. I went on my own. I thought it must be a mild infection and I'd be given antibiotics. While the doctor examined me he kept asking me questions: whether I had children, a boyfriend, whether I wanted more children. I was bemused; I thought he was just being inappropriate. He then left the room for quite some time. A nurse was looking at me. I got dressed and chatted to her. I still wasn't worried. The doctor returned and started shuffling papers on the desk and then said, "What do you think it is?" Still nothing registered with me. Then he leaned over the desk, held my arm and said, "I'm sorry to have to tell you this, but you have cancer". In retrospect I realize he was very sensitive and didn't know how to tell me. I remember saying, "Well, how did I get that then?" After that nothing went in. He mentioned hysterectomy, not being able to have children . . . but it was all a jumble, I was stunned. I was to go to the hospital the next day. There was nowhere to go. In the end one of the nurses saw how distressed I was and left me to sit in her office, where I cried for about an hour. I had so many questions, I even wandered back into the doctor's room but he was with someone else. It would have been so much better if I could have had someone with me to answer questions and somewhere quiet to cry and collect my thoughts. I didn't want to upset people in the waiting room.'

Sheila felt confused during the interview. She thought that the doctor had tried to tell her the bad news in a sensitive way, but that he could have done it a lot better. She also needed longer with him afterwards, somewhere to cry, and more time to take in the information and to ask questions.

The manner in which news is broken can influence a person's ability to cope with the implications of the news. If it is done badly, the recipient may well experience unnecessary distress; conversely, if it is managed well, the person is likely to trust the health care system and feel supported. All health care workers are likely to have to impart bad news at some time, be it the results of a blood test or the diagnosis of an illness.

Table 5.1. *How to break bad news*

Be prepared.
- Plan so that plenty of time is available.
- The person giving the news should know the woman or couple and have the necessary knowledge.
- If the woman is with a partner, friend or relative, then they should be included if she wishes. Ask her who she would like to be with her.
- Plan what are the main things you need to say.

Giving the news.
- Explain clearly the purpose of the meeting.
- Explore the woman's expectations and knowledge about the situation; the giving of information should follow from this discussion.
- Listen carefully and try to be relaxed. Do not hurry; try to match the woman's mood.
- The news should be given simply and clearly, avoiding jargon; technical terms should be explained. Initially, the test result or diagnosis may be enough.
- Give the woman or couple time to take in the news.
- Accept that strong emotional reactions may result and that these are normal in the situation; do not try to stop them.
- Be empathic and enquire about feelings if they are not expressed.
- Be honest and answer questions that are asked.
- Be supportive by listening and acknowledging distress.

Ending the interview.
- Let the woman/couple know how much time you have left.
- Repeat and summarize the information and the implications that you have discussed.
- Make sure that an early follow-up appointment is arranged, so that further questions can be answered and concerns addressed.
- Discuss what the woman or couple wish to do immediately after your interview; they might want the opportunity to sit in a quiet room for a while, to have a drink, or to arrange for transport home.
- Communicate to relevant staff, for example, in the clinical notes, what you have told the patient.
- After the interview give yourself some time to relax.

Laura was six months pregnant and on holiday in Scotland when her waters broke. She went to a local doctor.

'You don't take it on board; it was unreal. I didn't think I was going to go into labour. We went for a walk and I assumed everything was fine.'

She described the consultation.

'As he examined me, he looked worried. He did an internal examination. It never occurred to me that the baby may have died because she was so active. The thing that I found most difficult was he said I must come and sit down. I said I want to get my husband (who was outside) *and he said no, come and sit down. I didn't question that. He sat across a huge desk. He told me that there was a lot of fluid, he didn't know what it was and that we needed more sophisticated tests to find out. I needed to be in a specialist unit and the nearest one was on the other side of Scotland.*

I went outside to sit and wait with Phil (her husband). *I was anxious but still thought everything would be alright. The doctor came out and as he passed us in the waiting room he said, "There is a possibility that they could save the baby". Then I just went to pieces.'*

Sometimes, as in this case, a definite answer may not be available. Nevertheless, most people appreciate being told the truth; this can be followed by discussion of possible courses of action. It is also worth remembering that a natural reaction to bad news is not really wanting to believe it. It can be helpful to prepare the woman, or couple, using a hierarchy of general to specific statements. Mary's baby was born prematurely and had respiratory distress syndrome. Her doctor (D) came to see her a few hours later.

D: Well, how are you?

Mary: *I haven't seen the baby yet, where is she?*

D: When she was born she was a bit poorly and we're looking after her in the special care baby unit.

Mary: *What's wrong?*

D: Some babies, especially if they are born early, haven't produced enough of a certain substance to enable their lungs to work properly. So we are helping her to breathe on a machine called a ventilator.

Mary: *Oh.* (Pause.) *How bad is it?*

D: It is difficult to say at the moment. She is still quite ill but we hope that she will come off the ventilator in a few days, if there are no other complications.

Mary saw the doctors regularly and had counselling sessions with the ward social worker. In this way she could absorb the information and the changes in her baby's progress from day to day.

In these situations further discussions and follow-up appointments are crucial because of people's tendency to deny unpleasant information, and also because distress and anger often render processing of the implications of the news inadequate.

Preparation for Investigations and Minor Operations

Anticipation of diagnostic investigations and minor operations frequently combine concerns about the actual procedure as well as anxiety about its outcome. For example, however routine the experience of a vaginal examination, a cervical smear test or antenatal ultrasound scan might be for the health care worker, a woman is commonly faced with important questions about her health as well as an intimate and sometimes uncomfortable procedure.

Clear information should be given systematically before such interventions explaining their purpose, the procedures involved and what a woman might expect to experience. Without this information (and, unfortunately, it is not always given), she is not in a good position to make a clear choice about whether she might want to undergo the procedure or not. Information giving is not a one-way process but rather an active interchange between two or more people. Good communication is more likely to happen when the woman or couple are regarded as being in a partnership with the helper, rather than being the passive recipients of expert knowledge. Explaining the reasons for actions and procedures in advance, is a way of enhancing people's sense of control.

Ideally, the following information should be discussed before an intervention takes place, in written or verbal form, or both:

- The name and purpose of the intervention.
- When and where it will take place, and its duration.
- Who will carry it out.
- Whether preparation prior to the intervention is necessary (for example, drinking water prior to ultrasound scan).
- What will happen during the procedure.
- How the woman might expect to feel.
- How she might best cope with any discomfort.

- Any possible side-effects or consequences (for example, vaginal discharge following colposcopy) and what they mean.
- Who will discuss the results and when they will be available.

Any questions should be discussed before the procedure takes place. Although some information sheets and booklets are available for certain interventions, it is usually helpful to tailor the information to suit your particular situation.

During the intervention it can be reassuring if you comment briefly on what you are going to do next, leaving full discussion of the outcome until afterwards. Usha recalls an internal examination.

'He explained what he was going to do first then during the examination he was quick and confident. I wanted to get it over with and didn't want him to slowly explain everything again. He did say, "This might be a bit uncomfortable, but it's nearly over". That was fine.'

Knowing what to expect can allay unnecessary anxieties and can encourage the woman to make use of her own coping strategies. Jill describes how she coped with the egg donation stage of her IVF programme.

'I knew how long it would take. I'd rehearsed it in my mind beforehand so that when it was happening I tried to imagine the eggs and used some breathing exercises.'

Relaxation (see Appendix B) and distraction can be useful methods of dealing with stressful or uncomfortable interventions. However, it is helpful to enquire whether a woman already has a preferred way of coping. Breathing exercises can provide a focus for relaxation and calming thoughts. Distracting images such as a mental picture of a relaxing scene, for example, floating in a pool or lying on a beach, or active thoughts about something unrelated to the procedure can be rehearsed beforehand. The woman can also discuss with a partner or relative what she wants him/her to do during the procedure. Obviously, these methods are more relevant if the intervention is perceived as stressful, if it is likely to cause pain or discomfort, or if the person anticipating the intervention is very anxious. Open questions eliciting fears, expectations and concerns can help to identify those who might need extra help.

As well as offering information about procedures and the sensations that might be experienced, it is important to inform women about their choices and the implications of these. Most will want to know the options available and many are unaware that they have choices.

For example, many women do not realize that they have the option whether to have prenatal screening tests. These tend to be presented as part of normal routine practice, and some women do not even know whether they have had the tests or not. The way information is given can influence the woman's decision, especially if the health care worker involved communicates his/her assumptions about what is best for patients. Helping women and couples to assess options and to make their own decisions are important skills which are relevant

---

Table 5.2. *Helping people to make informed choices*

First help the woman to feel confident that she has a choice; that it is her right to decide to opt for a treatment or test or not. Then assist her in going through the following stages:

Gathering information about options.
- What are they? What are they likely to achieve? Are there possible side-effects?
- Sources of information: health professionals, research findings, other women, self-help groups, books and leaflets. You can actively help the woman to have access to such information, but be aware of your own views and biases.

Processing the information.
- Think about and talk over the options and the implications of their outcomes in the woman's particular case.
- Look at the advantages and disadvantages of each option and how she feels when imagining each option.
- Do the interests of others conflict with those of the patient? The views of relatives and close friends are often sought when making difficult decisions.
- Is the woman concerned about the outcome if she does not follow the advice she has been given?

Making a choice.
This is often a balance, the best of two or more options. When facing a difficult decision, mixed feelings are inevitable and there is likely to be uncertainty whatever the decision. The woman can be prepared for this. The main thing is that she makes the decision that, after rational consideration, feels best for her. The helper can usefully make information available and act as a sounding board for discussion of the options. It can also be helpful to suggest that the woman takes more time to think, if the decision evokes strong conflicting feelings.

to those facing surgery, abortion, hormone and other treatments. If you do not know the answer to a particular question, it is better to be honest (rather than hazard a guess) or refer the person to see someone who has more specialist information or expertise, for example, to a genetic counsellor, a menopause clinic, an appropriate self-help organization, or for a second opinion.

Preparation for Surgery

There is now consistent evidence that preoperative anxiety is associated with postoperative anxiety, as well as postoperative pain and recovery. Women's fears and uncertainties when facing major gynaecological surgery were described in Chapter 2, and the need to inform them fully is now generally recognized, but not always systematically carried out.

The first step is to find out what the particular practices and procedures are in your health care setting. For example, several people might be involved in provision of information at different stages. Ideally, detailed information is given by the surgeon at the time that the decision is made about whether to have the operation. The general practitioner or gynaecologist will offer information which can be usefully supplemented with leaflets and recommended reading. It is better for information to be repeated than omitted, so whatever your role, you can try to make sure that the woman anticipating surgery has the opportunity to discuss: the decision to have the operation and alternative options; the nature of the operation; when it is likely to take place; the length of hospital stay and estimated recovery time; any concerns or anxieties; the expected personal impact of the operation.

I have come across one hospital that offers a pre-hysterectomy group meeting, following referral and prior to hospitalization, where women can discuss their concerns, receive information about the operation and its consequences, and discuss problems that might arise. These meetings are an economical and excellent way to offer information in a supportive setting. However, for most women such services are not available, and for those who would not attend, preparation usually takes place on admission to hospital. This is unfortunate because being admitted to hospital is a stressful time and the woman can easily feel overloaded with things to remember, and be less likely to retain information because of anxiety. Provision of information in categories and in verbal and written form, with breaks and opportunity for discussion, can help to overcome these problems. Preoperative information can be divided into five main categories:

Information about the ward. For example, where to find the telephone, bathroom and the nurse's office, the names of the staff and their roles and details of visiting times.

Information about the procedure. This is best given chronologically with the main events summarized. A leaflet is very useful for the woman to refer back to, as is a diagram of the operation. Information should be written simply, and should include details such as whether dressings, drips and drains will be used, as these can cause anxiety if not anticipated.

Information about the expected experience and sensations. This can include both physical and emotional reactions. You can describe, for example, how she might feel on waking, or when she begins to move about, and the possibility of feeling low after the anaesthetic.

Ways of coping. When discussing procedures and sensations, it is helpful to reassure by explaining the reason for the procedure as well as suggesting ways of coping with sensations, such as ways of getting out of bed. Discussion of methods of controlling postoperative pain should be included as well as the need for postoperative movement and exercise. (Liaison with a physiotherapist is advisable.)

Information about recovery. She will need to know about the necessity of resting, when she can lift objects, drive a car, resume sexual activity, and about follow-up appointments. It is difficult and undesirable to give exact times to begin activities but general guidelines are helpful, taking into account the person's fitness and health. It is useful to inform about symptoms or signs that might occur which would require medical attention. Some women might want to know about the availability of self-help groups (see Appendix A).

The different categories of information listed above may have differential effects. For example, Ridgeway and Matthews (1982) found that procedural information about surgery increased knowledge and satisfaction, while suggestions for coping (offered in a booklet) had most effect upon recovery, assessed by use of analgesics and reports of pain.

Giving information is best viewed as a dialogue and eliciting concerns is as important as putting across the information you have. It is not possible, however, to prepare someone for every eventuality so general statements such as, 'most women . . .', 'usually . . . but not in all cases', are helpful. Details concerning recovery can be referred to briefly before the operation, but discussed in full afterwards.

Most people will want to know about the ward. However, some, probably a small number, may not want to know about details of the operation and the sensations that they might experience. It is essential, therefore, that patients have the option to decline information without being made to feel ungrateful or difficult. Some people use denial and do not actively seek information; this can work in acute situations if anxiety is at a mild to moderate level.

In view of the common situation in hospital wards where time is limited and patients are interacting with many different staff, it is crucial to facilitate communication between staff by noting who has communicated what to the patient, and any personal concerns or requests she might have. It is best to have a key worker who can develop a closer relationship with the woman and who can be in a better position to discuss concerns and provide information, and repeat it as needed, during her hospital stay. Monitoring a woman's anxiety and concerns before and during hospitalization can alert staff to those who might have particular problems and who might want to take up counselling after surgery.

For further details of procedures and experience of hysterectomy, see Savage (1982) and Webb (1989). Support groups are listed in Appendix A.

Support Before, During and After Childbirth

Antenatal classes are now a standard provision for most women in developed countries. By giving information about pregnancy and labour, health workers and voluntary groups aim to increase knowledge and confidence and decrease anxiety about labour and child care. The focus tends to be predominantly upon pregnancy and the actual labour, leaving some women less certain about child care. This may be partly because it can be difficult to absorb all the necessary information, or to see beyond the hurdle of labour. Hospital and community classes are often available, and the content is variable, but usually includes the following:

• information about pregnancy, self care and physical changes;
• information about labour and childbirth, especially signs, stages and the physical process;

- methods of pain relief and information about medical interventions;
- relaxation, breathing and pelvic floor exercises to carry out before and during labour;
- group discussions and questions;
- a visit to the labour and maternity wards;
- information about early days after the birth;
- postnatal exercises (for example, abdominal, pelvic floor);
- breast and bottle feeding;
- returning home and caring for the baby.

In a recent study comparing hospital and community classes, both types of preparation increased knowledge and confidence about coping with labour and in caring for the newborn. The community classes also facilitated the development of friendships between participants (Hillier and Slade, 1989). Given the importance of social support in preventing postnatal depression, community-based classes would seem to have an advantage. However, continuity of care is valuable and hospital classes offer the benefits of being able to get to know the setting and the staff.

Antenatal classes can serve to remind women of their options and provide information about the reasons for events taking place and how they might cope. The use of a birth plan can help to enable women to express their wishes and to enhance their feelings of control over the birth process. Most hospitals provide a booklet giving information about the hospital routine, what to bring and visiting hours. If information about the procedures and their medical implications is provided, a woman will feel that she is participating in decisions both during pregnancy and labour.

Being informed about procedures and the process of labour can help women to prepare for how they might deal with the variety of situations or events that might occur. Again a key worker system is ideal so that there can be continuity between pre- and postnatal care, and so that the woman can discuss her concerns with the same person. The doctor and/or midwife who are present during labour are in a much better position to help if they have taken time to talk with the woman beforehand about her feelings, preferences and worries. Information and support are very much appreciated during labour as well, especially if things are felt to be going wrong or if she is feeling out of control. For example, Noel (see page 29) pointed out,

'When things started to go wrong I felt abandoned emotionally . . . you think you're not doing it right. It's then that you need more support and explanation.'

It is common for a woman to blame herself and feel helpless and depressed if her cervix is not dilating quickly enough or if she is not producing enough milk. These concerns require reassurance and awareness that women vary considerably. Even in an emergency a member of staff should try to give brief details and support, leaving full explanation until afterwards. Again skill is needed to convey the available options without a woman feeling that she should or ought to follow a particular suggestion.

After the birth, a midwife or doctor who delivered the baby might offer the mother/couple the opportunity to discuss the labour and birth. This debriefing helps to make sense of the experience and to follow up any additional queries.

Several variants of childbirth preparation have been carried out offering differing degrees of social support and counselling in an attempt to increase psychological well-being and reduce the likelihood of postnatal depression. For example, the National Childbirth Trust in the UK offers breast-feeding counselling, pre- and postnatal support, postnatal social meetings, baby-sitting circles and clothes sales. Postnatally health visitors are in a very good position to offer support and explore and clarify problems – ideally they try to meet the women in the antenatal period as well.

Additional counselling can be made available for women selected by antenatal screening (using criteria that predict postnatal depression; see Elliott, 1989) or by postnatal screening for depression (Holden *et al.*, 1989). Group support before and after the birth or individual counselling sessions by health visitors have been found to reduce depression. However, once again, the woman should feel able to decline the offer of help without feeling guilty or uncomfortable.

Brierley (1988) gives a very good description of a cognitive-behavioural approach to helping women with postnatal depression. Nicholson (1989) has developed a counselling approach in which mothers are helped to deal with the sense of loss arising from unmet expectations, as well as changes in social role and identity.

Pregnancy Loss

The past ten years has seen a welcome increase in the support and information available for helping people to deal with pregnancy loss. The grief process is now generally acknowledged, as are the specific difficulties in coping with the loss of a baby (see page 43). Parents are more likely to have the opportunity to hold their dead baby, keep a memento and arrange a funeral, factors which can help reduce the sense of unreality. Indeed, there is evidence suggesting that women who have had contact with their baby after her/his death are subsequently better able to face the death and cope with grief (Kirkley-Best and Kellner, 1982).

In 1991 the Still Birth and Neonatal Death Society (SANDS) produced 'Guidelines for Health Professionals' (Henley and Kohner, 1991), which has been endorsed by the Royal Colleges of Nursing and Medicine. This booklet is essential reading for anyone working with women who have experienced pregnancy loss.

Central to the guidelines is the need for information, good communication and support. Information and support are interrelated and necessary at every stage; for example, for those who know that their baby has died but who have to proceed with labour, for those who are dealing with grief, to those who are uncertain about practical procedures such as funeral arrangements. In order to help couples through this very difficult time, it is essential that support and information are provided in the context of a helping relationship or partnership; that is, a relationship characterized by respect, empathy, humility and genuineness. These qualities, which are described in detail in Chapter 4, are necessary for the helper to understand what the person or couple is going through, to listen and attend to what they are saying and feeling, and to know how and when to make choices available and to offer information. Ideally, a key worker will form a close relationship with the woman or couple. However, the person who delivers the baby is often seen to be very important, because she/he has experienced the loss with the parents.

Grief reactions are described briefly in Chapter 2, and ways of helping people to deal with distress in Chapter 4 are also relevant here. Helping bereaved people involves:

- Creating a relationship of trust, by being genuine, respectful, and engaging the person in a partnership, rather than an expert relationship.
- Giving people time to talk about whatever concerns them, and following their lead.
- Listening and being available so that people can go over what has happened several times, bring up new concerns, or simply be silent if they wish.
- Enabling the person or couple to express their distress freely by listening, demonstrating empathy and accepting that their reactions are normal. Resist the urge to *do* something; it is much more helpful to be with someone in their suffering.

- Helping them to explore what has happened and the implications for themselves, in their own time.

More information about bereavement counselling can be found in Parkes (1978).

As the events surrounding the loss and the reality of the loss sink in, parents understandably have many questions to ask. The information that is commonly needed can be divided into several different types:

- Practical information about what has happened, why it has happened and what may happen next.
- Information about medical procedures and ward practices.
- Information about arrangements concerning registration of the death, funerals, memorial ceremonies, burials and cremations.
- Information about common emotional reactions – that these are intense but normal, permissible and part of the grief process.
- Information needed to enable choices to be made. Most couples will be unaware of options and choices, so care is required in presenting possibilities in a sensitive manner.

Information should not be given all at once, in one interview. Instead, listen to the parents first; they are likely to ask you questions in their own time. Find out what they know and think already. The guidelines about giving bad news, discussed earlier in this chapter, are relevant here.

When helping a couple in this very difficult situation, it is necessary to avoid assumptions and not be judgemental, and to take account of personal circumstances, beliefs and reactions. It is usually best to give information to both parents (if there is a partner) and to be available to answer questions, to repeat information, and to go over discussions a number of times. If you go to see a parent and she does not want to talk, it is important to respect her wishes; it does not mean that she will not want to talk at another time.

Painful information is hard to take in, and when a person is in distress, information will be forgotten. As mentioned already, information should also be given in written form, in the appropriate language. Time is needed for couples to consolidate information, to understand their experience and to begin to grieve. Couples should not feel pushed or pressurized and will probably need several opportunities to make decisions, for example, about whether or when to hold the baby.

Most parents are pleased that they have held their dead baby and many regret it if they do not have the opportunity. However, facing the pain is difficult for parents and staff, and the desire to avoid the death and the baby is a normal reaction. In view of this, staff have to tread a delicate path, encouraging and not pressurizing, if necessary returning to make the offer again later. For example, Veronica (midwife) went to talk to Anne after the death of her son. Veronica held the baby.

Veronica (looking at the baby and stroking his face): *Would you like to take him now?*

Anne: *Oh I don't know.* (Cries.) *He looks so perfect . . .* (Is comforted by her husband.) *I don't know. It would upset me too much.*

Veronica: *There's plenty of time . . . most women feel like that. Part of you wants to, but it feels really hard. It is not something you have to do, but most women who do are pleased afterwards . . .*

Anne strokes the baby's face and cries.

Veronica (after staying for a while): *You don't need to decide now . . . Would you like me to come back later?*

Anne: *Yes that will be fine.*

Later Anne and her husband held the baby and Veronica offered them time on their own with him. Veronica demonstrated how to speak with respect, as well as giving information and options.

Laura works as a clinical psychologist with couples dealing with pregnancy loss. She has herself lost two babies and describes her experience after her daughter Jessica died.

'I was terrified to hold her. Phil (her husband) *had held her first. He gently but firmly encouraged me to hold her. It is hard and scary but so important. I held her for a while and gave her back. They* (the staff) *didn't tell me about dressing her or her care. Now I wish I could have done more for her, but at the time I didn't realize that I could.'*

Making options available is a skill. For example, parents need to know that they can keep a memento, but this does not have to be a photograph; it can be a lock of hair, a name band, a footprint, etc. The main message is to give parents information about the range of options and permission to feel free to make their own choices. This is especially the case when choices are based upon religious and cultural beliefs and practices which differ from those of the health worker.

Good communication between staff is essential to avoid misunderstandings and unnecessary distress. For example, new staff at follow-up should know that a woman has lost a baby from her medical notes. Care should be taken to avoid medical terms such as 'second trimester abortion' which, if communicated to the patient, devalues her personal sense of loss.

A dilemma often voiced by health staff working with people who have lost a baby is how to behave. Is it appropriate for me to cry? How much time should I allocate for practical care? Is it my job to sit and listen? I have no doubt that to listen and spend time with grieving parents is one of the most helpful things that health care workers can offer. You may feel some conflict between your professional role and the natural human urge to respond to suffering. To be overly professional is likely to be perceived as uncaring; to be busy and avoid the grieving parents is not helpful. Some expression of feeling by staff is valued and appreciated by parents and seen as a sign of caring. Laura describes how her nursing sister related to her.

'She was very good. She was sympathetic but not anxious about approaching me. You need someone to be strong for you, not being uninvolved or detached . . . Being sad for you, but also not feeling overwhelmed by it. Someone who recognizes the intensity of the feelings. At that time the midwives who were there during the delivery and afterwards are the most important people in your world. They have been through it with you . . . they've had the relationship with you and the baby.'

Staff support and training is crucial in order to help midwives and other health care workers to deal with the problems they face in their contact with death and bereavement.

Good communication, provision of information and support is extremely helpful for parents. In these very sad circumstances, more regular counselling can be offered as an option before the parents go home. Some may not want to take this up, some may seek support from voluntary groups such as SANDS, which offers an excellent network in the UK, and some may want to take up the offer at a later date. In a study carried out in Oxford (Forrest *et al.*, 1982) parents who were offered extra support and counselling by social workers or midwives were less likely to be clinically depressed at 16 months after the loss, than a group who received no extra support. (Refer to the case of Jen in the next chapter for an example of counselling after pregnancy loss.)

Summary

❑ Women repeatedly express the need for information and support in obstetric and gynaecological practice.

❑ Information and support should go hand in hand; information being provided in the context of a helping relationship, which is characterized by respect, genuineness and empathy.

❑ Before giving information, it is important to explore the person's knowledge, expectations and concerns.

❑ Information should be provided simply and clearly, avoiding jargon. Answer any questions, repeat key points, summarize, and check that you have a shared understanding of what has been discussed.

❑ Information-giving should be seen as a dialogue. Do not overload the person. Instead, take time to listen and respond to questions and reactions.

❑ When giving bad news, it can help to be prepared by planning what you want to say and making adequate time available:
– the person giving the news should know the recipient;
– the information should be given simply, as described above, and preceded by a discussion of the person's understandings and expectations;
– be supportive by demonstrating empathy, listening and acknowledging distress;
– the interview should end with a definite plan for the future, such as a follow-up appointment, and consideration of the person's immediate needs for support.

❑ Ways of providing information and support before investigations and interventions are described. These include clear discussion of the reasons for a woman's decision to have the investigation, her expectations and any fears or anxieties she might have, the purpose of the investigation, how she might prepare for it, how she might expect to feel, any possible side-effects, how she might cope, and how and when the results (if any) will be communicated.

❑ People are not always aware that they have choices about whether they need to have certain procedures performed or not. Helping women to make informed choices involves discussing the available options, making information available, and discussion of the advantages and disadvantages of the options and their implications.

❑ Preparation and support for women undergoing major surgery, childbirth and those dealing with pregnancy loss are described in detail, based on the principles of helping and information-giving discussed here and in the previous chapters.

6

New Perspectives and Problem-Solving

The previous two chapters were concerned with exploration and understanding of the person's problem, and providing information and support in acute settings. This chapter deals with helping people to find appropriate solutions to the problems they have identified. For some, this might mean gaining new perspectives on their difficulties with the benefit of information. For others, it might involve gradual lifestyle changes, or more subtle shifts in attitudes, or ways of coping with more chronic problems. The stories of Carol, Janet, Jen and Pauline are continued to illustrate a variety of counselling approaches.

The chapter begins with a discussion of ways of challenging existing models, or providing new perspectives on problems. Problem-solving skills (setting goals and making changes, Egan's stages 2 and 3), assertiveness, and stress management skills are described. The chapter also looks at ways of maintaining changes, as well as how and when to bring counselling to a close. It ends with a discussion of how to help people to deal with the health care system, and the role of health promotion in obstetrics and gynaecology.

New Perspectives and Alternative Models

The very process of exploring a woman's model of her problem can help to shed fresh light upon it. By encouraging her to verbalize thoughts and feelings and to consider the implications of her model, she is likely to begin to question its validity herself. Moreover, the awareness that she is valued might, in turn, increase her sense of self-worth, so that she feels able to tackle her problems with increased confidence.

In Chapter 4, ways of checking common understandings were described, such as making empathic statements and summarizing. Once a shared understanding has been achieved, the next step in helping the person to find solutions to problems, is to work with them to assess the validity of the model, and to consider new perspectives or alternative ways of understanding the problem. This is not to assume that a different model or explanation is necessarily more appropriate; it may be that the original model is felt to be the most useful after having considered the alternatives. Before examining the validity of existing models, there are a few general guidelines to bear in mind:

• New perspectives should be very tentatively introduced, in the context of a trusting relationship, so that the woman seeking help feels free to accept or reject ideas that are discussed.
• Before offering alternative explanations or ideas, prime the woman so that she can see that there are likely to be several ways of understanding most problems.
• People often seek one reason to explain their problems; in fact, most problems have a number of causes, which usually interact.
• The aim is to find a model of the problem that is most helpful to the person seeking help.
• Be aware of your own biases and beliefs, and be explicit about the models that you are discussing.

The initial model can be gently challenged by offering information. We have seen how this commonly occurs in acute situations, when diagnostic information is given. Information also can be helpful in attempting to understand the cause(s) of more chronic problems. In obstetrics and gynaecology, problems such as chronic pelvic pain, premenstrual tension, and depression during the menopause, are often difficult to understand. It is important to be as informed as possible about these issues. (An outline of the main issues and research findings can be found in Chapters 1 and 2.)

A common tendency, particularly when people are seeking help from doctors or health care services, is for them to adopt a purely biological model to explain their problem, and to neglect the role of psychological, social and cultural factors. For example, many people understandably believe that pain signifies disease, and that there is a one-to-one relationship between pain and bodily damage. A more complex model of understanding the factors that influence and maintain pain might be introduced by discussion of the gate control theory (see page 40 for further details). Similarly, reproductive processes that involve hormonal changes, such as menstruation, childbirth, and menopause, tend to be regarded as causing emotional problems. Again, psychosocial causes, such as life stresses, bereavements, social problems and lack of fulfilment, are often neglected; for most women distress arises, or is exacerbated by, what is happening in their lives (see Chapter 2).

It can be helpful to point out how social structures, such as idealized views of motherhood or negative images of older women, can constrain women's natural expression of thoughts and feelings and can undermine self-esteem. Over-conformity to restrictive gender roles often contributes to depression, and women's subordinate position in society can give rise to much personal distress. Increasing a woman's awareness of the impact of psychosocial factors can empower her to feel able to make changes, rather than to blame herself, or her body.

Mary came to see me because she was feeling depressed and irritable before her period; initially she wanted medication to regulate her cycle. She explained how her moods were affecting her marriage, and how she made every attempt to prevent her husband from knowing how she felt. She spent the days at home doing housework and taking her three children to different schools and various social activities. Having worked before her children were born, she had always intended to return but could not envisage how to do this now. She admitted that she felt unfulfilled, but maintained that she should not bother her husband with her problems and strove to put on a brave face. Most of the time she succeeded in this. However, before her period she found that it was much more difficult. She became irritable with her children and took to bed in the evenings to avoid having an outburst with her husband. Gradually she began to acknowledge that the core problem was more likely to be her dissatisfaction with her lifestyle and her own unmet needs, rather than being entirely hormonal. Discussion of her beliefs 'that she should be happy in her current situation', and 'that her husband would disapprove of her pursuing her interests', enabled her to attribute some of her distress to her situation and to make plans to make changes in her attitudes and behaviour.

It is important to discuss new perspectives, or possible explanations tentatively, and to avoid direct challenge of a person's understandings, especially if this is based on limited information. A common mistake is automatically to attribute a person's problems to psychological factors because they have had emotional problems in the past. Karen was angry and upset after she had been to see her doctor because of abdominal pain. She had been sexually abused as a child and had suffered from intermittent depression during the past four years. 'She listened to me for a while and then said that it was probably psychological'. Karen's pain may well have been influenced by her mood. However, confronting her with this interpretation without discussing a range of possible explanations was perceived as rejecting and unhelpful.

When beginning to look at alternative models it is best to be open-minded; be prepared to reassess your own thoughts together with the person. As discussed earlier, you will need a clear understanding of the person's view of the problem and its implications. It is often helpful to give examples to illustrate how psychosocial factors can interact with physical ill-health. In the case of pain, you could discuss how pain is usually more tolerable when one is actively engaged in, or distracted by, a pleasant or absorbing activity. A more powerful way of pointing out situational or psychological influences is to comment, in a tentative way, upon how a woman experiences the symptom during the interview. For example, one woman I saw described her pain as being constant at quite an intense level. As she talked about her problems she became tense and held her abdomen, where the pain occurred. Towards the end of the session I showed her some relaxation exercises and she noticed that when she was more relaxed, the pain was reduced. Comparison of the effects of the two mood states upon her pain helped her to acknowledge the influence of non-biological factors.

Keeping a diary is another way of helping people to see the links betwen their symptoms and situational factors. This can be done simply, using a chart with days along one side with a rating of the severity of the symptom (on a 0 to 5 scale) next to each day. Space should be left for comments so that the person can make a note of anything particular that they were doing that day, or what was happening at the time that the symptom occurred. The inter-relationship between symptoms and events can be examined and can be used to provide evidence in support of, or against, a particular model. This is, for example, a useful way to understand the nature of menstrual changes, and the influences upon mood across the cycle.

Other ways of assessing the value of new perspectives or explanations include:

- discussion with the helper;
- discussion with other people;
- trying out new ways of behaving and noting the results.

Rachel, for example, believed that she was an incompetent mother. An alternative explanation was considered, namely, that her mothering was as good as most other people, but that part of the problem was her tendency to self-criticism. Following discussion of what she was actually doing with the baby, and her attendance at a postnatal support group, she learned that her feelings were not so unusual and that, in comparison with others, she was doing quite well.

Exploring different perspectives can, in itself, be a very helpful process in reaching solutions to problems. There is some overlap between this process and the problem-solving skills that are discussed in the next section.

Problem-Solving

Once a problem has been identified, and the best possible understanding of its causes and influences achieved, help might be needed to make specific changes, for example, to lifestyle, relationships, or to ways of coping. As well as helping someone to find solutions to a particular problem, the aim here is to demonstrate or teach a way of approaching problems that might be applied to situations in the future.

Egan (1990) provides a detailed account of the steps that can be followed to help people to tackle problems; these include setting clear aims and goals, planning action, implementing plans and evaluating the outcome.

Setting goals

Help the woman to clarify her aims, that is the general changes she wants to make, and then encourage her to set realistic, specific goals that are consistent with these aims and her value system. This can be done by discussion of what she thinks and feels would be an acceptable target, and consideration of possible pressures from others. She should set herself goals that she wants to reach, as opposed to those she feels she ought to reach. It might be necessary to weigh up the pros and cons of different goals by listing the positive and negative implications of each. Goals can also be listed in order of priority.

Goals need to be realistic. In other words, they should have enough impact upon the problem to be worth carrying out, but not so difficult that they are unlikely to be achieved. They need to present a reasonable challenge. If the overall aim requires major changes, then it is helpful to set a series of goals to be tackled within a realistic time frame. Consideration of possible obstacles to their achievement, and discussion of the impact of achieving the goal upon the person's life, can help to assess whether the goal(s) are realistic or not. Some people find it helpful to imagine having achieved a particular goal, and to describe what it would be like.

Goals need to be defined specifically, and in detail, so that it is clear when they have been achieved. For example, one woman decided that, in order to manage her pressured lifestyle, she needed more time for herself. However, she found this difficult to do when the goal was defined so generally. In contrast, she was able to achieve the more concrete goal of having an hour to read on her own, every evening, between 6 and 7 o'clock.

Planning action and implementing changes

A person can be helped to think creatively about a range of ways of achieving the goal. Encourage her to 'brainstorm' by writing down as many possible strategies for action as she can, without judging the suitability of the options. You might facilitate this process by asking about how she dealt with similar problems in the past, or encouraging her to think about how different people might respond. It can be useful to make this process explicit so that the woman feels that she is learning a skill that is applicable to other situations. Separating the creative stage from the evaluation of the options encourages clear thinking and a positive approach to problem-solving.

Next, each option can be examined in turn and evaluated as to its likely outcome. This would involve consideration of the advantages and disadvantages, and possible risks and benefits, of each plan of action. The woman should then be helped to choose the best-fit plan and decide on the action, or series of actions, needed. Actions might be graded across a time course, so that each stage is implemented only when the previous one has been achieved. For example, Kathy wanted to be more assertive at home and at work. She decided that her first goal would be to say no to her children when they made demands upon her while she was eating. When she felt comfortable about doing that, she intended to move on to goals related to her partner and, after that, tackle goals related to work. Some people might need to learn new skills, such as stress management or assertiveness skills, in order to achieve their goals. Others might need to seek information and advice, for example, about alternative child care arrangements or employment.

Before putting plans into action, it is best to think through with the person any possible difficulties that might occur, and how they might be overcome. Changes need to be consistent to a large extent with the woman's belief systems and chosen way of life. When making changes, practical issues such as work, time, distance to travel and the views of family and friends, need to be considered. Both obvious and subtle barriers to continued change need to be explored. For example, Pam was approaching the menopause and decided to engage in regular physical exercise and a yoga class in order to help herself to reduce stress and keep in shape. However, because she had not made other changes within the systems around her, the new activities became rather punishing.

'I started going twice a week to keep fit and one evening a week to yoga. It was great but the housework started to mount up. Bill and the kids made their usual demands. I'd come back from yoga to chaos . . . honestly it's defeating the object . . . I'm even busier than before.'

Pam was helped to put her case assertively, and household tasks were shared more evenly, enabling her to enjoy the benefits of her classes.

Relationships can serve to encourage or reinforce certain behaviours that maintain problems. For example, a woman who is anxious about going out alone, might be accompanied everywhere by her husband. He may think that he is helping, but is, in fact, maintaining the problem. He may even be content with the current situation at one level. In this example, changes in his reactions to his wife's increasing independence would need to be explored. Similarly, people with chronic pain are often encouraged by their families to be inactive, when, in fact, graded activity is very helpful.

Once a plan of action is decided and the woman is prepared for possible problems that might arise, the helper can offer support and encouragement, by praising successes and helping her to tackle any further difficulties.

Evaluating the outcomes

Monitoring progress and evaluation of each strategy is part of the process of change. However, it can be helpful to have a particular time to consider the impact of the attempted changes, and whether goals have been reached. The woman herself should be encouraged to evaluate her own progress, and helped to engage in reasonable self-criticism, as well as self-reward.

Consideration of outcomes, and a realistic appraisal of the reasons for a particular outcome, can be a useful exercise, because this understanding is likely to influence subsequent attempts at change. For example, some people, if their attempts are thwarted, attribute the negative outcome to themselves and feel helpless. However, others might accept little responsibility for a lack of achievement and blame other people or external events. Neither of these extremes is likely to reflect the reality of most situations. It can be valuable to consider, with the person, those factors over which they have some control and those which are relatively uncontrollable, and to discuss strategies to deal with such events. On the other hand, some people have difficulty in acknowledging their own role in achieving positive outcomes, and might feel that the helper deserves all the credit. It is obviously important in this situation to point out the person's strengths and endeavours that enabled change to take place. It is equally important to learn from mistakes and, with honesty and humility, the helper can be open about his/her oversights and formulate new or modified plans with the person.

Assertiveness and Stress Management

Stress management and assertiveness skills are relevant to dealing with life's problems and are as important for health care workers as they are for women seeking help. Frequent monitoring of stress and giving priority to one's own emotional and physical well-being are highly recommended. (Ways of reducing stress are outlined in Table 6.1 and relaxation exercises in Appendix B. See also Burnard, 1991.)

Stress management and assertiveness skills can be taught individually or in groups (for example, self-help groups), or as part of staff training. Groups have several advantages in that rehearsing different situations and giving feedback is easier, and support and encouragement are more readily available.

Women often are aware that they have difficulty dealing with angry feelings, and are not assertive enough. Being unassertive means not being able to ask for what you want or need, not valuing your own worth or rights, agreeing with people to make them feel comfortable, and putting everyone else's needs before your own. Conversely assertiveness means being able to express your wants, needs and feelings appropriately, and being effective in relationships and in work situations. (See also Dickson, 1982.)

Assertive people communicate self-respect and a wish to have their own needs met, while respecting others. Assertiveness entails constructive criticism and negotiation rather than submission or domination. It does not mean bullying or losing one's temper. Being assertive includes the ability to express positive as well as negative feelings. The following questions will help you to assess how assertive you are:

- Do you have difficulty in saying 'no' to persuasive requests?
- Are you overly apologetic?

- Can you correct someone who has misunderstood you?
- Are you able to complain if you feel badly treated?
- Do you value and express your own opinion?
- Can you express and receive affection and compliments?

Assertive behaviour includes non-verbal as well as verbal messages. Situations can be practised or rehearsed in pairs, or in threes with one person observing. The following components should be addressed:

- eye contact: maintain reasonable eye contact
- tone of voice: speak loudly enough to attract attention
- facial expression: if you are saying something serious, look serious
- posture: sit or stand firmly, don't cower
- emotions: a simple, clear, unambiguous message is best, without undue qualifications or excuses; repeat firmly if necessary.

Constructive group feedback and discussion about the appropriateness of ways of behaving in different settings can provide useful additional learning.

Table 6.1. *Managing stress*

- Understand the nature of stress; the physical, emotional, cognitive and interpersonal results of stress.
- Learn to recognize personal signs of stress.
- Acknowledge stress and take some responsibility for reducing it.
- Examine perceptions of situations and events. Stress often results from a feeling that the demands of a situation cannot be met by one's abilities or resources. However, one's appraisals of situations and perceptions of demands and one's ability to cope may not be accurate.
- Discuss ways of coping with stress. Some approaches are more helpful (for example, take time to think, talk to a friend, take a relaxing bath, make plans to reduce workload, tackle a problem at work using the appropriate channels) than others (for example, smoke more, eat a lot, ignore the problem, panic or 'catastrophize', bottle things up, blame others).
- Use problem-solving skills to assess what changes can be made and their implications.
- Instigate positive changes that are likely to have more than temporary effect.
- Learn ways of relaxing and exercising to reduce the impact of stress.
- Give priority to a healthy lifestyle.

Case Studies

Before going on to discuss ways of maintaining changes and how to end helping relationships, the stories of Carol, Janet, Jen and Pauline are continued here, in order to give some sense of the kinds of changes that can be facilitated.

Carol

Carol initially sought help because of premenstrual tension (see pages 35 and 75). She had begun to acknowledge that she felt unhappy about her life and that these feelings were more acute before her period. She lived alone, was rather socially isolated and felt that she had underachieved. She said that she felt rejected by her parents. After exploration of her expectations, her own theories and psychosocial situation (see page 75), she met again with Sister J. (SJ) who had arranged regular supervision for herself with a clinical psychologist in the hospital.

Carol's general aim was to be free from PMT and to go back to college. Before agreeing a contract, this goal had to be made more specific. A problem-solving discussion centred upon models of understanding PMT, how Carol currently coped with her distress and the necessary steps and hurdles that had to be overcome before she might be in a position to go back to college.

Carol: *Well if I think about it, I do have these feelings the rest of the month.* (She had been talking about being anxious about making changes and lacking confidence.) *But before my period I feel like giving up. I've no energy . . . so I suppose I tend to swing from having some positive plans to nothing at all. That's when I drink more, so I suppose that makes me worse and less in control.*

SJ: *So you go from one extreme to the other. It looks to me as though your thoughts about yourself might vary a lot too.*

Carol: *At PMT times I think I'm a failure – I'm hopeless . . . That's what my parents used to say about me . . .*

SJ: *. . . And at other times?*

Carol: *Well, sometimes I do think I'm not too bad . . . I'm not stupid and I think I could do well at college.*

SJ: *And how are you feeling now?*

Carol: *I feel fairly positive . . . I've taken one step by coming here I suppose.*

SJ: *Yes you have . . . let's think about what you will need to do to reach your long-term aim.*

With help Carol specified the following initial goals that would be needed in order to work towards her long-term aims.

1. To cope with thoughts and feelings more effectively in the week before her period.
2. To use relaxation when she felt tense and to limit her use of alcohol.
3. To be able to go out shopping or to the library without undue anxiety.

She acknowledged that her current expectations (that she should be able to go to college), heightened her feelings of failure. She began to see that by setting herself specific and realistic short-term aims, which were possible to achieve, she might be able to see herself as someone who could succeed. She negotiated a contract with Sister J. to work on these three aims, which were made more specific still.

1. To monitor thoughts ('I'm a failure', 'I want to give up', 'I feel good about myself') and feelings (anxiety, energy) during the menstrual cycle.
2. To learn to relax as a way of reducing anxiety.
3. To challenge her overly negative self-perceptions.
4. To limit alcohol to, at most, one or two glasses of wine (with meals) each day.
5. To set herself graded daily tasks involving going out to places in order to increase contact with other people (for example, going into local shops to buy a paper). She wanted to be better informed and to feel more confident in daily social interactions.

It was agreed that it would be helpful for Carol to monitor her thoughts and feelings in a diary for a month before tackling the other aims. Six weekly, one-hour sessions were arranged after the monitoring period to work on the short-term aims. Carol agreed to attend the sessions and was reasonably confident that she would be able to try to achieve each goal, but was concerned about how she would feel before her period. Progress would be reviewed after six weeks.

Carol rated her moods according to (1) how anxious she felt and (2) how energetic she felt, on a zero to ten scale in her diary every day. She also monitored the frequency of particular thoughts. This needed to be carried out simply by making a tick in her diary each time she thought 'I'm a failure', 'I want to give up', and also when she had positive thoughts about herself such as, 'I think I can overcome my problems'. She also noted her days of menstruation and any activities or events that occurred, as well as her alcohol intake.

From her diary recordings, Carol noticed a pattern in which her mood had fluctuated during the past month, but found she was not especially more anxious or less energetic premenstrually. She had felt particularly anxious and negative about herself following a chance meeting with an old school friend in the street, who asked Carol about her life. Carol felt envious and inadequate in comparison. The diary helped her to understand the relationships between her mood, life stresses, thoughts and menstrual cycle.

She became more aware of her negative thoughts, or self perceptions, and began to question their validity. She recalled that the feeling of being hopeless and a failure began because she compared herself with her brother, who she felt was favoured; she had never really questioned the assumption that she was less able.

Several sessions were spent discussing the diary and setting graded goals such as increasing social contact and activities. Relaxation was used when she felt tense and before her period, and ways of limiting her alcohol intake were discussed. It became clear that, rather than helping, the alcohol exacerbated her negative moods and premenstrual headaches.

By keeping a diary and making some changes, Carol could see that her initial theory about her distress (that it was mainly due to PMT) was not very helpful to her. Although she did feel a bit more tense before her period in the second month of the monitoring, she found that she could cope with the feelings. Talking about her negative self-concept and challenging her sense of failure by achieving small goals, increased her confidence.

'I'm keen now to read and find out what I'm good at. Before, I think I was so desperate to go to college because that was my family's expectations – I didn't think that I might want to do my own thing.'

Carol now felt reasonably confident about going out. It seemed that it was partly envy and fear of being seen as a failure, evoked by social comparisons, that led to her feeling tense in social situations, rather than her being phobic of the situations themselves. Reviewing her progress led Carol to the following new aims:

1. To apply for work in a library.
2. To find out about courses in typing and word processing.
3. To enrol in a relaxing evening class, such as yoga, drawing or pottery.

In addition, Sister J. arranged to see her for six-monthly follow-up appointments to monitor her progress.

Janet

Janet came to see me because of her pelvic pain. Her story is described on page 18 and explored further on page 75. Although her pain had been present for several years, it had become much worse since she witnessed the death of a friend in a road traffic accident. She had been unable to share her grief because of her feelings of guilt and because her family did not encourage such discussions. It appeared that her parents were able to support her when she expressed her distress in terms of physical pain, but they felt uncomfortable with and avoided facing raw emotions.

A shared theory about the pain was established, based on the gate control theory (see page 40). Because Janet's grief and conflicting feelings about her friend's death were very much the focus of her distress, the following aims were agreed:

1. To meet for four weekly sessions, followed by four fortnightly sessions (Janet was changing her working hours after the first month) to allow time for Janet to talk about and understand her feelings about her friend's death.
2. To monitor her pain daily during this time (noting down the intensity of pain on a zero to five scale in a diary) and to learn relaxation exercises to help her to reduce the tension she felt in her pelvis.

The sessions were essentially non-directive. Janet spoke of the actual accident in detail and about what she felt she could have done. She described her friendship, and was encouraged to remember the difficult as well as the good times. Further information about the grief process (see page 44) helped her to feel that her reactions were not abnormal. At the end of each session Janet practised relaxation and was encouraged to keep her diary.

Discussion of her grief led to consideration of her upbringing, and an attempt to understand why her parents made her feel that feelings should be suppressed.

'That's how they always were; if I was upset they'd say, "Come on, nothing's broken". Mum's a bit anxious and Dad tries to prevent anything worrying her, I think. I know that her parents died when she was in her teens or twenties but they don't talk about it.'

She began to talk to one or two other friends about her grief and felt reassured that they seemed to understand. In one session she became very angry about the accident, but also with her parents and myself.

Janet: *How can I accept this; it could have happened to me. It's as if I'm the only one that's reacting. Why aren't you all angry? Don't you care either?*

MH: *You want people to see that what happened and your feelings matter.*

Janet: *I mean sometimes I think, if I'd had the accident, would they have cried?* (Cries.)

MH (pauses): *Perhaps they might react like you . . . holding it all in but feeling bad inside . . .*

Janet: *Yes, I suppose . . . maybe . . . we were all doing the same thing.*

Between the fifth and sixth session Janet had talked to her mother about the accident.

'I was quite surprised when I told her. She said that she thought I was feeling bad, but that she assumed that I wanted to be left alone. I had a bit of a cry with her . . . honestly, I'm 24 years old . . . but we feel a bit closer now.'

During the last session we reviewed progress. Janet's mood had improved and she was feeling more relaxed at work. Her tension was being eased by relaxation. The pain was still there in the background, but became worse when she was menstruating and when she was very tired. She felt that she could manage the pain better, for example, by pacing her activities, using relaxation and gradually broadening her social life.

'I'd like to see how I manage on my own now. I want time to develop my social life. The girls at work are always asking me to go out with them, so I will do that – but gradually.'

We agreed that she contact me in six months to let me know how she was. I also let Janet know that she could contact me if she felt she really needed to in the meantime.

Jen

Jen's problems also involve grief, but the focus for her was being able to deal with the panic evoked by thoughts of her baby who died shortly after birth seven months before (see page 47). She had begun to talk about the loss in exploratory sessions (see page 77) and had had the experience of 'surviving the strong emotional reactions'. She agreed to meet her doctor (D) six times and then review progress. Jen was concerned about being upset after their meetings, so sessions were arranged so that she would have some time to relax afterwards, and at a time of day so that she would not have to return to work. The following goals were agreed:

1. That she would like to be able to get used to talking about Thomas (the baby) and the events surrounding his death during the sessions.
2. That she would aim very gradually to approach situations (in particular contact with friends and family) that she was avoiding for fear of being overwhelmed by intense feelings.
3. That she would include Dave in later sessions to talk together and understand each other's grief.

It was important to let Jen work at her own pace so a fairly flexible time frame was agreed for these goals.

During the first three sessions, she spoke freely and recalled in detail her pregnancy, the labour, the birth and circumstances surrounding the death of her baby, and her thoughts and feelings. She cried a lot but left the sessions having recovered. The important issues here seemed to be to follow her lead, accept her distress, and enable her to have time to recover before the end of the session (see page 80 for further discussion of dealing with distress).

'It's very hard, very hard indeed. I know I'll never really get over this, but in a way, although I'm getting all churned up again, it makes me feel in touch again. I'm alive.'

After the third session she was still having difficulty seeing her friend (who had a young baby) and her brother's family. She voiced her envy and anger in the next session; acknowledging these feelings made it easier to go and talk to her friend.

'In the end I phoned her and said what I feel like when I see her. That it's not her fault, but I find it so hard with the baby there . . . looking at me. She said she'd go out with me to see a film or something and Andy (her husband) *could babysit. That was thoughtful . . . I think I could do that.'*

Progress was reviewed at the end of the fourth session. Jen said that she could talk more easily about the baby in the meetings, and was beginning to feel less 'like a time-bomb', with friends and family. However, at home she felt that Dave seemed more withdrawn and she was aware of his reluctance to engage in conversation about her counselling or their loss. A meeting was arranged with the couple together. Dave was gently encouraged to explain how he felt. For example, he had felt guilty because he had not been fully involved during the birth and immediately afterwards (Jen had gone into labour early and unexpectedly).

Dave: *I've thought all along that you* (Jen) *hadn't forgiven me for not being there at the beginning. I felt so bad afterwards . . . it was too late though.*

D: *You feel that it's too late to help each other.*

Jen: *That's ridiculous really. You have been helpful to me . . . but at times I've wondered if you felt so bad, because you just cut off.*

Dave: *I've always handled things like that.* (Looks down.)

Jen (puts arm round him): *I know that really . . . that you do feel . . .*

D: *You both seem to be trying to deal with the hurt but in your own, different ways.*

Six more fortnightly sessions were arranged with the aims of supporting Jen and Dave and providing time where they could try to understand their differing experiences of grief.

Pauline

Pauline's experience of gynaecological surgery and the initial exploration of her postoperative feelings of distress are described on pages 27 and 78. Pauline had, to an extent, clarified her feelings by separating her anger about the poor communication surrounding the operation from her sadness about its implications. Initially, her main concern was about infertility and the effects this would have upon her future and her current relationship.

While she was in hospital, she had been unable to use her usual coping strategy of keeping busy and distracting herself by working very hard. In her family, and in the past, she was regarded as the 'strong successful one'; she looked after her sisters and brothers, but inside she felt somewhat empty and isolated. The operation and hospitalization brought new problems (infertility), but also highlighted the fragility of her usual way of coping with stress.

Six sessions were arranged to help Pauline to think about her ways of coping with distress and the effects these had upon her relationships. She was also aware that she was pushing her partner away because of her feelings about not being able to have children. She wanted to understand this because she valued the relationship.

In the first session Pauline spoke about why she felt so split inside (between the successful coping person and the empty, lonely one).

'I was the favourite at home. They all saw me as successful. You know, if anything went wrong . . . ask Pauline. I encouraged them all to stay on at school. But really they had no idea what I've been through.'

She talked about her childhood and the very difficult times she had with her 'aunt' in Jamaica.

Pauline: *Of course when I came to England I was so pleased to have a family I didn't really look back . . . I think my mother spoiled me really . . . you know, to make up for those years. The others* (her sisters) *were jealous. I wasn't that close to them, they kept their distance.*

MH: *So you felt unable to show how you really felt to your mother or your sisters?*

Pauline: *Well, yes . . . I mean not until recently. After last time* (first session) *I did talk to one of my sisters. I told her a bit about what it was like for me.*

In the next session she talked about her relationship with her partner.

Pauline: *He really irritates me. I don't really want to be touched. Like this morning, he started cuddling me in the kitchen . . .*

MH: *Can you say what you thought and felt at that time?*

Pauline: *Don't come too near . . . well it might have led to sex.* (Their sexual relationship had stopped since the operation.) *I suppose I don't want him to get too close. What's the point of having sex if you can't have children. I know he says he doesn't mind but I think one day he'll decide he wants children and . . . where will I be?*

MH: *So you think he might reject you in the future because you can't have children.*

Pauline: *You can't tell what's going to happen anyway, I know. There are good things about the relationship. I don't want to make any big changes at the moment and he seems happy as things are. He knows I don't want sex yet and that's OK – but I think I do reject him in other ways . . . like giving affection . . . which must hurt him.*

As the sessions continued, Pauline began to talk to her family more, and as a result she felt that their understanding of each other had increased. During one week she felt particularly low and lonely and she missed the next session.

'*When I feel bad like that I just want to be on my own . . . to go to work . . . come home and keep busy.*

We discussed Pauline's expectations about change and ways of dealing with distress. She had felt a failure because she was keeping busy and had not wanted to come to the session. It was necessary at this stage to clarify goals. For example, the aims of counselling were not to change her coping strategies completely, but to help her to be more aware of them and to use them more flexibly. Specific situations (from work and at home) were discussed in a problem-solving manner in an attempt to explore various ways of coping and their implications.

At the end of the six sessions Pauline still felt fairly vulnerable and low at times when she thought about her infertility, but she felt more at ease with herself and had opened up communication with her family which, in turn, had made her feel more understood.

'I feel less split . . . more easy within myself. I can admit to feeling bad and I do let Ben (her partner) help me. I still feel upset about the operation. I probably wouldn't have had any more children but . . . it's something that time will heal. I still keep busy, but I feel less desperate and driven than I did before.'

Maintaining Changes

A woman's contact with health care workers (in obstetrics and gynaecology) is likely to have fleeting impact relative to the influences of her past life, other current problems and her psychosocial situation. The non-expert or mutual-participation relationship (see page 50) gives those seeking help responsibility for decisions, thereby avoiding an undue dependence. The helper can usefully take an increasingly passive role in problem-solving, leaving the woman the space to formulate plans herself, in a sense as a rehearsal for dealing with future life changes.

As discussed earlier, changes are more likely to be maintained if they are reinforced in the person's environment. Sometimes adjustments need to be made in relationships with others. For example, Janet and Pauline talked to their families about their perceptions and feelings, and Jen considered it important that her husband joined the counselling session to enable him to understand her grief as well as his own.

In some situations a friend or partner can be engaged as a helper; for example, to encourage and support someone who is dealing with a chronic problem; or to remind her to carry out plans and monitor progress in problem-solving; or to help her to cope during a medical intervention. An intimate relationship or close friendship can often provide this type of invaluable support.

For those who are more isolated, part of making and maintaining change, or having a more fulfilling life, might be to begin to develop a social network. People's needs vary, however, so it is important not to impose one's ideas about lifestyle upon others.

Support groups and self-help groups are sought by many women and can provide regular meetings as well as information and advice. Some deal with particular reproductive problems or events, while others offer support and help with more general life and relationship problems, such as bereavement, alcohol or physical abuse (see page 137). Health care workers need to be aware of, and liaise with, such groups in the community. They also might usefully help women who wish to set up their own groups, if there is a perceived need. Details of UK organizations and charities, women's health groups and other services are listed in Appendix A. Social groups will suit some people but not others. Riordan and Beggs (1987) offer some useful criteria for helping people to find the group that is right for them.

When and How to End Counselling

For most health care workers contact with patients is dictated by their role in the health care system. Some nursing staff, for example, see people while they are in a hospital ward and are unable to follow up on them as out-patients. Time constraints and demands upon a service frequently limit the number of out-patient counselling sessions or visits that can be offered.

It is essential to have a strong framework in which to work: where your role is clearly defined; where you know where to go for advice, supervision or support; and where there are clear boundaries or limits to your input. A common mistake is to respond to someone's distress by taking on an overly caring role, being available at all times and thereby encouraging dependence, rather than self-reliance. It is equally important to recognize when you do not have the skills or time available to meet someone's needs. For example, for some problems, change is best maintained by group support, or you might find that there is a marital problem that a colleague is better equipped to deal with. These decisions can be difficult, and supervision, together with a referral network, is recommended.

The duration of the helping relationship is also determined by the nature of the person's problems. For example, learning to live with grief following a stillbirth is a long-term process, as is dealing with a chronic illness. However, counselling prior to surgery or finding ways to reduce anxiety in pregnancy, may require briefer contact. It is also necessary to be able to recognize severe psychiatric disorder (for example, if someone is very depressed and feels unable to cope, or appears to have thoughts or beliefs which are not based in reality), so that the appropriate help can be provided. Once again seek advice or supervision if you are unsure.

The approach outlined in this book, focusing primarily upon communication, counselling and problem-solving skills, generally involves short-term input. By agreeing on an initial number of meetings, with an inbuilt review, both the person seeking help and the helper can be prepared for a time-limited relationship. Egan (1990) put the helping relationship into perspective when he said that people should be encouraged to find and use the resources from their everyday lives to manage problems and to develop their unused opportunities. Long-term relationships belong in people's everyday lives, not in helping encounters.

Of course, some people will drop out, or prematurely terminate their contract. One way of trying to prevent this is to discuss motivation, concerns and barriers to attendance when making an initial contract, and to establish realistic expectations. This is clearly more the case when patients come to see you regularly in a hospital or clinic setting, as opposed to brief contracts when information is offered; but even for one-off meetings one's role needs to be defined.

Reviewing and evaluating progress at the end of an agreed number of meetings can result in several outcomes:

- An additional number of sessions might be arranged with the aim of working towards a redefined goal.
- A decision may be jointly made to bring the process to a close.
- Follow-up meetings may be set up to monitor planned future changes and their maintenance.

Obviously, patients and health care workers might want to terminate the meetings unilaterally for different reasons, such as lack of motivation, achieving some change which has relieved acute distress, or the helper might think that the work has been done even though the patient disagrees. Again clear discussion of aims and expectations, anticipation of difficulties and close monitoring of progress help prevent these situations. However, at the end of the day, the person's wishes and decisions need to be respected.

If ending is built in as a natural part of the contract, it is less likely to be perceived by the other person as a rejection. This may be potentially more of a problem for some people, for example, those who have experienced early loss or who have problems in relationships. It is equally important to be aware of one's own reactions to endings; for example, if someone has been particularly interesting and rewarding to work with, it may be difficult to see letting go as a positive step. It can be helpful to decide with the person, early on, what degree of progress or change would be sufficient for ending the helping relationship. In addition, a final review of change and future plans can make the ending positive.

Dealing with the Health Care System

Most people can benefit from increased knowledge about the health care system and how to negotiate it, and all health care workers can help people to obtain such knowledge. A frequent complaint is being unaware of choices, such as whether procedures are optional, whether there are alternative treatments, or whether they are entitled to a second opinion. A woman's wish for a cognitive map or total picture of the people involved in her care, and their roles, should be accommodated.

Anxiety, ill-health and diffidence about asking questions frequently interfere with good communication. Some people may be helped by rehearsal of an important interview, for example, or by drawing up lists of questions, or by assertiveness training. Relaxation and self-talk can be used to help others to reduce anxiety prior to an appointment. In some cases people may need help to understand how they can give feedback if they have particular complaints.

Some people have unrealistic beliefs about what health services can offer. Doctors especially can be seen to be imbued with life-giving and godly powers. Dissatisfaction frequently results from over-dependence upon doctors or expectations that they can perform miracles. These situations can be avoided to some extent by including a woman in her treatment as much as possible and by acknowledging errors, the limits of one's level of skills or, for example, lack of consensus in scientific research. It is often lack of attention to patient's human needs, for example, not listening or showing respect or empathy that is at the basis of complaints. But it is easier to complain about tangible mistakes than qualities in a relationship. Complacency and acquiescence to poor communication and poor services should not be encouraged. For example, Margie threw in this remark after telling me about her experiences in an antenatal clinic:

'I felt like a piece of meat, moving from one place to another. Looking at all those despondent women's faces, being made to wait . . . I don't know, what can you expect . . . Doctors will never really know what it's like. They're always on the other side.'

It is up to women like Margie to give constructive feedback.

Health Promotion

There are many opportunities for health promotion in obstetrics and gynaecology in health care settings. The term health promotion is used here to include:

- information about health;
- information and advice about health problems;
- assessment of personal health risks and lifestyle;
- discussion of ways of reducing health risks and improving health and well-being.

Antenatal care, or preparation for childbirth, at its best meets most of these aims, particularly where groups continue postnatally and offer training in relaxation, physical exercises and general discussion about life with children, as well as child care.

Obvious examples of health education (a narrower term usually referring to the provision of information) include information about contraception, breast-feeding, cervical screening, breast self-examination, mammography, hormone-replacement therapy, immunization, smoking, diet and exercise. Leaflets of this type are available in most clinics and hospitals. However, it is now recognized that, in order to have impact upon health-related behaviours such as smoking and exercise (or lack of it), more than knowledge is usually required. Barriers to change include lack of motivation, inability to set graded realistic goals, lack of support, costs, time and many others. Groups set up to deal with specific problems or health issues are usually more effective than information alone for those who choose to try to make lifestyle changes.

Health promotion groups might be usefully made available to women attending family planning, well woman or screening services, or to women reaching a particular life-stage. For example, in an ongoing study, the author, with Karen Liao, is evaluating a primary care service for 45-year-old women in five general practices. The aim of the service is to prepare women for the menopause and beyond, by offering group sessions covering the following areas:

- Discussion of beliefs, myths and concerns about the menopause, and ageing and health during midlife.
- Providing information about the menopause (biological, emotional, social and cultural aspects).
- Discussion of lifestyles including healthy diet, exercise and stress reduction. The need for calcium and weight-bearing exercise to help reduce the risks of osteoporosis in later life is included as is

discussion of cardiovascular disease and breast cancer – problems that are of concern to older women.

- Information and discussion about how to deal with hot flushes and night sweats, of hormone replacement therapy (risks and benefits) and how to help oneself.
- Group discussion of lifestyle, emphasizing the differences between women and the choices available.
- Problem-solving and goal-setting: women are encouraged to set themselves a personal target aimed at improving their health and well-being. For many this is to engage in exercise (such as brisk walks, swimming, dancing), for some it means taking time off for themselves after a demanding day, others aim to increase social activities or to change jobs.

For further information about preparation for the menopause see Hunter (1990), and Hunter and Coope (1993).

While focusing upon individual change, health promotion also needs to address broader social and political issues. For example, change might be impeded by lack of community facilities for women, or by women's fears of going out alone at night. Similarly, sensitivity is needed to respect the differing values and priorities of individuals.

There is some overlap between health promotion groups, which are more likely to be short-term and specific and led by a health care worker, and self-help groups which tend to offer information as well as sometimes providing longer term support. Self-help groups also serve as a means whereby women can collectively express their needs and recommend changes to their health care systems at local and national levels.

Such services, however, tend to attract more women from white, middle-class backgrounds. In order to make health promotion available to different community and ethnic groups, and sensitive to their needs, intensive publicity and liaison or outreach workers may be needed to work within local community networks. See the Ethnic Health Factfile (Karmi, 1992) for more information and useful addresses.

Summary

❑ This chapter deals with helping people to find solutions to problems in less acute settings.

❑ New perspectives and alternative ways of understanding problems should be explored tentatively, in the context of a trusting relationship.

❑ In general, the role of psychosocial factors is often neglected in models of reproductive problems, and the complex influences upon them not given due emphasis.

❑ However, it is important not to act on assumptions about the causes of someone's problems before discussing in detail her model, the evidence for and against this, and possible alternatives.

❑ The validity of different models can be examined by providing information, discussion, using examples, monitoring the relationships between symptoms and situations or events, and by noting the outcomes of changes in behaviour.

❑ For some, clarification of the cause(s) and support may be enough; others might need specific help in knowing how to tackle the particular problems they face.

❑ Problem-solving skills include the following: setting clear, specific, realistic goals; planning and implementing changes (by assessing barriers to goals, benefits and the skills required) and offering support and encouragement; evaluation of the outcome(s), discussion of the likely reasons for these outcome(s) and a review of what has been learnt.

❑ Assertiveness training and stress management skills, including relaxation training, are valuable skills to help patients and staff to deal with life's problems and to improve effectiveness.

❑ Changes can be best maintained by setting realistic goals, by being aware of the impact of change upon the person's relationships and environment, by discussion of possible future problems and by helping people to find support in their locality.

❑ Decisions about how and when to end counselling are made easier if the initial aims are clearly specified and if the helping relationship is one of shared responsibility.

❑ People can be helped to deal with the health care system by increasing their knowledge and understanding, by giving constructive feedback, and by being given the opportunity to ask questions and to play an active part in their treatment.

❑ Many opportunities exist for health promotion in obstetrics and gynaecology, ranging from leaflets being made available about particular health problems, to groups being set up to help people to support each other through change.

Conclusions

This chapter covers evaluation, training and supervision – key issues for those working in health care and helping roles. But first a brief summary of the conclusions so far will be presented.

Principles of Communication and Counselling

- Dissatisfactions with health care services concerned with reproductive problems result from inadequate information, misunderstandings, insensitivity, lack of control over decisions and treatment, and discontinuity of care.
- Communication skills, involving careful listening (about symptoms as well as the person's theories and beliefs), empathy and exploration, in the context of a relationship of respect and mutual participation, are needed to improve interactions between women and health care workers, and to prevent unnecessary distress.
- Information and choices need to be made available. Assumptions about a woman's problems, needs or lifestyle based on beliefs about her culture, race, ethnic group, sexual preference, religion, age or social class should be questioned and challenged.
- Counselling should be patient-focused with the helper's and patient's roles clearly defined within a particular time-frame. By arranging links with community resources, adaptive changes are more likely to be maintained.
- Helpers (or counsellors) who arrange regular counselling sessions, or health care workers who are having to cope with difficult problems such as infertility, pregnancy loss or cancer in day-to-day work, require peer or staff support and supervision. Further training is recommended for those who wish to increase their skills.

Evaluation of Counselling

Ongoing evaluation of change and progress when working with patients has been described in Chapter 6. This is built into the problem-solving approach advocated in this book and is made possible by clear definition of aims and goals. Monitoring progress can be relatively straightforward if goals are fairly concrete, for example, cutting down on smoking or alcohol intake, undergoing a procedure that previously evoked undue anxiety or taking fewer painkillers.

However, in many cases the aims of counselling may not be so tangible or so closely linked to behavioural change. When the aim is to look at cognitive and affective (emotional) reactions, various measures can be used. These can be general measures of mood, for example, the Spielberger State and Trait Anxiety Scale (Spielberger *et al.*, 1970) or the Beck Depression Scale (Beck *et al.*, 1961). In addition specific rating scales can be developed for your own needs. For example, if you wish to examine the effects of relaxation and graded activity upon the person's experience and reactions to pain, you may want to measure several variables (see examples of rating scales below). Your particular intervention may differentially affect the pain ratings.

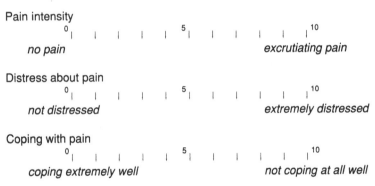

Pain intensity

no pain   excrutiating pain

Distress about pain

not distressed   extremely distressed

Coping with pain

coping extremely well   not coping at all well

Examples of pain rating scales

Diaries are useful for monitoring the effects of an intervention, as well as for understanding temporal relationships between changes made (for example, relaxation practice) and experience of the problem (for example, depressed mood, anxiety, pain, PMT or hot flushes). A baseline recording of a particular aspect of the problem will enable you to examine the effects of counselling. If applied in this way, the evaluation is a product of the joint involvement of the patient and the helper.

When questionnaires are used in evaluation it is advisable to encourage the person to be honest and to overcome the wish to give socially desirable responses in order to please you. However, measures should not overload or be too intrusive.

Giving mutual feedback at the end of counselling by reviewing what was helpful, the nature of change and the perceived reasons for change can be beneficial for all concerned. Evaluation of services should be seen as a central part of clinical practice, and action research (finding answers to practical clinical questions) is a basis on which to plan counselling input. For example, I recently began working in a unit providing services for infertile couples. Before taking referrals, we agreed to initiate team meetings and to carry out a survey of patients' perceived needs for different types of counselling, such as one-to-one contact, support groups, one-off 'open-door' discussions. This survey guided subsequent input.

Effective help in obstetrics and gynaecology

There are many examples of effective application of communication and counselling skills to obstetrics and gynaecology, and several have already been described in the preceding chapters. Provision of information prior to surgical intervention has been found to reduce postoperative anxiety and pain reports, with detailed information yielding better results (Wallace, 1984). However, type of information can be tailored to achieve differing outcomes (Ridgeway and Matthews, 1982). For example, information about surgery may increase knowledge and satisfaction, while teaching cognitive coping strategies has most impact upon indices of recovery (analgesics and pain reports).

Applications of non-directive counselling to problems such as chronic pelvic pain (Pearce et al., 1982) have been shown to be effective. Counselling interventions can improve the outcome (assessed by measures of depression and general distress) for those who have experienced pregnancy loss (Forrest et al., 1982) as well as postnatal depression (Holden et al., 1989; Leverton and Elliott, 1989; Nicholson, 1989). Cognitive-behavioural treatments have been used to help anxious and depressed clients, those with chronic pain and those reporting premenstrual symptoms (Slade, 1989) with beneficial effects. The preliminary results of a cognitive-behavioural treatment for hot flushes experienced by menopausal women, suggest that this may be a useful approach.

In the evaluation of psychological therapies, not only is the symptom or presenting complaint assessed (such as frequency and duration), but also changes in other indices such as its impact on daily life, resulting distress and the woman's perception of how well she is coping with the problem. In general, counselling and psychological therapies help people to formulate a clearer picture of their problem and to develop adaptive ways of dealing with it. As a result, health psychologists and others are keen to explore more subtle changes by, for example, asking questions about people's causal attributions, their own theories and their coping skills (see Brewin, 1990).

Evaluation is also likely to become increasingly important if the case has to be argued that counselling services are cost-effective and beneficial in health care settings.

Support for Health Workers

Training, supervision and support should go hand-in-hand. The process of helping can be emotionally and physically draining, particularly if you work without support or a clearly defined role, or in an organization in which the value of psychological care is not openly acknowledged. Attempting to attend to people's emotional needs is likely to increase the helper' exposure to different issues and distress. If the working system is not able to provide the helper with the necessary support and supervision, the overall outcome may be negative, resulting in increased stress and possible resentment, high staff turnover and low morale.

It is now being recognized that nurses, at a young age, shoulder a considerable amount of responsibility and are faced with numerous difficult and distressing situations (Llewelyn, 1989). Stress can be alleviated by increasing the helper's personal resources and/or by modifying the nature and extent of the demands upon him/her. It is not uncommon for people working in caring roles to feel that their skills or emotional input are undervalued or underused, or are taken for granted. Isolation can be a problem for nurses and others working in community settings, and communication problems in large organizations can lead to unexpressed needs and concerns and lack of recognition. If helpers feel that the demands on them are excessive, poor communication may result, motivated consciously or unconsciously by the need to avoid further stress. To put this more positively, psychological care is most effective when staff feel they have been taught the skills and receive ongoing encouragement and supervision in their work.

Your work setting

In order to know where you can seek support and advice, you need to look at the structure of your work setting. Is it a hierarchy, with a pyramid of leaders and workers, or a chain of command with sections and subsections? Is it a team, working with a group of individuals or key workers, each accountable to other members of the team? Or it may be a network, consisting of a number of people, each with a leader but without responsibility towards any other individual or group within the network.

In hierarchies you would go to your supervisor for advice, while in a team this should come from other team members. Networks are less satisfactory, because there is less clarity about whom you can really call on for support. If you are in doubt about your position, talk to your colleagues. Find out how your organization functions. Are there clear channels of communication? Is it responsive to changing circumstances? Are systems arranged in the best interests of those they are set up to serve? Are short-term solutions sought for problems which require more extensive changes in order to make life easier?

Helping patients to help themselves and giving them the opportunity to be involved in their health care can put additional strains upon organizations. Such change, if it is to be successful, needs to be sanctioned and supported by those in charge. You need to know to whom you are accountable, who is responsible for your supervision and support, and who you can go to if you meet difficulties, if you have personal problems, or if you want to suggest changes to how the organization is functioning.

Training

Training and supervision can be viewed as a continuum. Group sessions or workshops focusing upon stress management or communication skills (using role-play) can provide excellent training in the workplace. These methods are included in some professional training courses, but unfortunately not all.

There is a wide variety of counselling courses available, ranging from short courses (one or two days) offering an introduction to specific counselling skills, to longer courses requiring full-time or part-time commitment and leading to a qualification in counselling. The choice can be bewildering.

The British Association for Counselling (BAC) runs short courses and provides information on training available in the UK. In their code of ethics they recommend that counsellors monitor their work through regular supervision with professionally competent supervisors, and that they are accountable to patients and colleagues for what they do and why. The Family Planning Association in the UK also runs short courses in counselling skills, and specific courses are available for those working with fertility problems and pregnancy loss (see Appendix A). Anyone employed as a counsellor in health care settings should undergo a recognized training; unfortunately, such training is not yet a requirement within the National Health Service.

If you wish to pursue a counselling career, it is advisable to seek a course that is set up by a recognized college or organization and one which makes available a full description of the course and the tutors. Do your own research by talking to ex-students and seeking personal recommendations. The British Psychological Society now offers a Diploma in Counselling Psychology which allows successful candidates to use the title 'Chartered Counselling Psychologist'. Prospective candidates need to assess postgraduate courses in counselling psychology against the criteria of the Diploma.

Training courses for particular types of psychological therapy exist, and include, for example, behavioural psychotherapy, cognitive therapy and various forms of psychoanalytic psychotherapies. Contact the British Psychological Society for further details, or the British Association of Psychotherapists. There are advantages, however, to courses that teach skills that can be easily applied in your work setting and that offer a conceptual framework which is consistent with regular supervision at work. Professional training as a nurse counsellor, clinical psychologist or psychotherapist requires a longer term commitment of between two and six years, and personal experience of therapy is essential for most psychotherapy courses and will usually be recommended if you are seeking a career in counselling.

Supervision

Supervision involves one person in a work setting acting as a support person for another. This should occur regularly, with fixed times set aside for the purpose. The supervisor's role includes:

- listening, reflecting back, clarifying and problem-solving;
- empathy and emotional support;
- advice and teaching;
- evaluation of goals and career development.

Supervision thus also requires good communication and counselling skills. Ideally, the content of a particular session should be negotiated at the beginning of that session, with the focus upon the person being supervised. The supervisor is often one's immediate superior. However, peer supervision is being increasingly used. Co-counselling involves mutual supervision of peers with two people meeting regularly dividing the time between them to take either the supervisor or worker role and then reversing.

Rehearsing situations and obtaining feedback in a supportive setting can increase both skills and confidence. Role play is a useful tool, and can be done in pairs or in trios. Having a third person to offer feedback to the two in conversation can increase learning. Criticism should always be constructive in that all feedback should be specific and phrased in a positive way. For example, 'You always speak too quietly', can be expressed as, 'You would appear more involved in this situation if you speak more loudly'. Make explicit the idea that everyone has skills to improve!

If a particular staff member has experience in counselling or psychotherapy he/she might take on the role of supervisor for several individuals. Sometimes an outsider (from another department or institution) can provide supervision. Supervision can also take place in groups. However, the focus and boundaries of the group need to be clarified and issues such as confidentiality about patients and one's own disclosures discussed.

If you are lucky there may be the opportunity for different types of supervision. For example, Anne works in a busy psychiatric ward. She has times to discuss the details of her work on the ward with her staff nurse, her academic work with her nurse tutor and she uses a ward staff group to let off steam resulting from day-to-day frustrations. Mala, a nurse working in an Accident and Emergency clinic had a less positive experience:

'A nurse who was doing research started a staff group to talk about stress on the unit. Some of us went along because there are really a lot of problems. It was helpful, but we found out later that one of our managers thought that we were going because we couldn't cope.'

When discussing personal needs it can be helpful to talk about stress in terms of demands and available resources for support in order to avoid 'blaming the victim'. Staff groups appear to be more successful if they are oriented around specific difficulties experienced at work (such as dealing with pregnancy loss), rather than focused upon the personal emotional problems of the members. Used in this way, and preferably led by an active task-orientated leader, they can be an effective means of reducing stress. Remember that support, supervision and good communication skills go hand-in-hand, raise awareness amongst your colleagues, and help develop an ethos in your work setting in which skills and needs as well as limitations can be openly discussed.

Look after yourself

Finally, it is worth remembering that in order to help others you need to look after yourself. Use the skills outlined in this book, for example, problem-solving, stress-management, assertiveness training and relaxation. Make sure that you take time off, that you work within clear boundaries and that the demands upon you do not exceed your personal resources or those of your work setting. For further information about how to deal with stress in health care settings, see Burnard (1991).

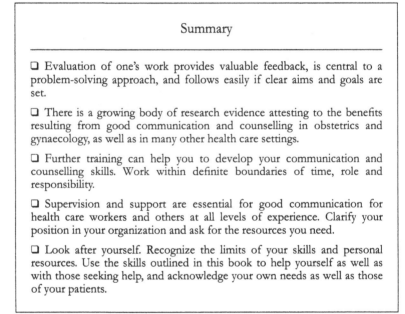

Summary

❑ Evaluation of one's work provides valuable feedback, is central to a problem-solving approach, and follows easily if clear aims and goals are set.

❑ There is a growing body of research evidence attesting to the benefits resulting from good communication and counselling in obstetrics and gynaecology, as well as in many other health care settings.

❑ Further training can help you to develop your communication and counselling skills. Work within definite boundaries of time, role and responsibility.

❑ Supervision and support are essential for good communication for health care workers and others at all levels of experience. Clarify your position in your organization and ask for the resources you need.

❑ Look after yourself. Recognize the limits of your skills and personal resources. Use the skills outlined in this book to help yourself as well as with those seeking help, and acknowledge your own needs as well as those of your patients.

Appendix A: Organizations and Support Groups

Association for Improvements in Maternity Services (AIMS) 163 Liverpool Road, London N1 0RF.

Association for Post-natal Illness, 7 Gowan Avenue, London SW6 6RH.

Association of Radical Midwives, 62 Greetby Hill, Ormskirk, Lancashire L39 2DT.

Birmingham Women's Counselling and Therapy Centre, The Uffculne Clinic, Queensbridge Road, Moseley, Birmingham B13 8QD.

British Agencies for Adoption and Fostering, 11 Southwark Street, London W1P 1HD.

British Association for Counselling, 37a Sheep Street, Rugby, Warwickshire CV21 3BX.

British Association of Psychotherapists, 37 Mapesbury Road, London NW2 4HJ.

British Infertility Counselling Association, 50 Middlethorpe Grove, Dringhouses, York YO2 2LD.

British Pregnancy Advisory Service, Austy Manor, Wooten Wawen, Solihull, West Midlands B95 6BX.

The British Psychological Society, St Andrew's House, 48 Princess Road East, Leicester LE1 7DR.

Brook Advisory Centre (for family planning and contraception advice), 233 Tottenham Court Road, London W1P 9AE and 2 Lower Gilmore Place, Edinburgh EH3 9NY.

Caesarian Support Network, 2 Hurst Park Drive, Huyton, Liverpool L36 1TF.

Cancer After-care and Rehabilitation (CARE) 21 Zetland Road, Redland, Bristol BS6 7AH.

Carers National Association, 29 Chilworth Mews, London W2 3RG.

CRUSE Bereavement Care, 126 Sheen Road, Richmond, Surrey TW9 1UR.

Cry-sis (support for parents of crying/sleepless babies), BM Cry-sis, London WC1N 3XX.

Down's Syndrome Association, 153–155 Mitcham Road, London SW17 9PG.

Eating Disorders Association, Sackville Place, 44/48 Magdalen Street, Norwich NR3 1JE.

Endometriosis Society, 245a Coldharbour Lane, London SW9 8RR.

Ethnic Minorities Advice Bureau, 1a Station Road, London SE25 5AH.

Family Planning Association, 27–35 Mortimer Street, London W1N 7RJ. 4 Museum Place, Cardiff CF1 3BG. 113 University Street, Belfast.

Foundation for the Study of Infant Deaths (Cot death research and support), 15 Belgrave Square, London SW1X 8PS.

Gingerbread, 35 Wellington Street, London WC2E 7BN.

Herpes Association, 41 North Road, London N7 9DP.

Hysterectomy Support Network, c/o 3 Lynne Close, Green Street Green, Orpington, Kent BR6 6BS.

ISSUE (National Fertility Association) St George's Rectory, Tower Street, Birmingham B19 3UY.

Lesbian and Gay Switchboard, Tel: 071 837 7324.

Meet-a-Mum Association (MAMA), 3 Woodside Avenue, South Norwood, London SE25 5DW.

Miscarriage Association, 18 Stoneybrook Close, West Bretton, Wakefield, West Yorkshire WF4 4TP.

National Association for Mental Health (MIND), 22 Harley Street, London W1N 2ED.

National Association for the Childless, 318 Summer Lane, Birmingham B19 3RL.

National Childbirth Trust, 9 Queensborough Terrace, Bayswater, London W2 3TB.

National Council for One Parent Families, 255 Kentish Town Road, London NW5 2LX.

National Federation of Self-Help Organisations, 150 Townmead Road, London SW6 2RA.

National Information for Parents of Premature Babies (NIPPERS), 49 Allison Road, Acton, London W3 6HZ.

National Osteoporosis Society, P.O. Box 10, Radstock, Bath, Avon BA3 3YB.

Pelvic Inflammatory Disease Support Group, c/o W.H.R.R.I.C. (see below).

Pre-Eclamptic Toxaemia Society, Eton Lodge, 8 Southend Road, Hockley, Essex SF5 4QQ.

Rape Crisis Centre, P.O. Box 69, London WC1 9NJ.

Relate: National Marriage Guidance, Herbert Bray College, Little Church Street, Rugby, Warwicks CV21 3AP.

Samaritans, 10 The Grove, Slough, Berks SL1 1QP.

Scottish Marriage Guidance Council, 26 Frederick Street, Edinburgh EH2 2JR.

Sickle Cell Society, Green Lodge, Barretts Green Road, Park Royal, London NW10 7AP.

Society to Support Home Confinements, Lydgate, Lydgate Lane, Walsingham, Bishop Aukland DL13 3HA.

SPOD (Association to aid the personal and sexual relationships of people with a disability), 286 Camden Road, London N7 0BJ.

Stillbirth and Neonatal Death Society (SANDS), 28 Portland Place, London W1N 3DE.

Support after Termination for Abnormality (SATFA), 29–30 Soho Square, London W1V 6JB.

Thalassaemia Society UK, 107 Nightingale Lane, London N8 7QY.

Twins and Multiple Births Association, c/o 41 Fortuna Way, Aylesby Park, Grimsby, South Humberside DN37 9SJ.

Women's Counselling and Therapy Service, 16 Harold Road, Shirley, Southampton.

Women's Health and Reproductive Rights Centre (W.H.R.R.I.C.), 52–54 Featherstone Street, London EC2A 3AR.

Women's Health Concern, 317 High Holborn, London WC1V 7NL.

Women's Therapy Centre, 6–9 Manor Gardens, London N7 6LA.

Appendix B: Relaxation and breathing exercises

A variety of relaxation instructions and tapes are available. Most combine muscular relaxation with breathing exercises (see Bernstein and Borkovec, 1973). The following is a shorter version, combining the systematic tensing and relaxing of muscles in the body, with attention to rhythmic, gentle breathing.

- Sit in a comfortable chair, with loose clothing and freedom from interruptions for about 15 to 20 minutes.
- Notice yourself resting in the chair – your muscles, the heaviness of your body and your breathing.
- Begin by tensing your arms and hands by making tight fists and holding your arms tight for a few seconds. Then let them drop loosely . . . Notice the feelings in the muscles and feel the relaxation spreading down from your shoulders to your fingertips.
- Now raise your shoulders, taking a deep breath, push your shoulders up and back. Hold it . . . and relax. Let your shoulders, arms and hands rest and become heavy and feel yourself resting back as if it would be an effort to move.
- Notice your breathing – it should be gentle, even, passive breathing from your stomach (not from your chest). Just feel the air passing gently across the back of your throat . . . and each time you breathe out you will feel heavier, calmer and more deeply relaxed.
- Tense your stomach, taking a deep breath, by making the muscles tight. Hold for a few seconds and relax.
- Repeat tensing then relaxing legs and feet, by stretching them out in front of you.
- Enjoy five to ten minutes at the end just relaxing and following your breathing. Imagine a peaceful scene if you can . . . feeling the sensations of the sun, sand and water, for example.
- Practice three to four times a week and you will learn to relax more quickly and deeply.

References

Areskog-Wijma, B. (1987) The gynaecological examination – women's experiences and preferences and the role of the gynaecologist. *Journal of Psychosomatic Obstetrics and Gynaecology, 6*, 59–69.

Bains, G. K. and Slade, P. (1989) Attributional patterns, mood and the menstrual cycle. *Psychosomatic Medicine, 50(5)*, 469–476.

Beck, A. T., Ward, C. H., Mendelson, M., Mock, J. and Erbaugh, J. (1961) Inventory for measuring depression. *Archives of General Psychiatry, 4*, 561–571.

Bernstein, D. A. and Borkovec, T. D. (1973) *Progressive Relaxation Therapy: A Manual for the Helping Professions.* Illinois: Research Press.

Beyenne, Y. (1986) Cultural significance and physiological manifestations of menopause: a biocultural analysis. *Culture, Medicine and Psychiatry, 10*, 47–71.

Bourne, S. (1968) The psychological effects of stillbirths on women and their doctors. *Journal of the Royal College of General Practitioners, 16*, 103–112.

Brewin, C. R. (1990) *Cognitive Foundations of Clinical Psychology.* UK: Lawrence Erlbaum Associates Ltd.

Brierley, E. (1988) A cognitive-behavioural approach to the treatment of post-natal distress. *Marce Bulletin, 1*, 27–41.

Briscoe, M. (1982) Sex differences in psychological well-being. *Psychological Medicine Monographs Supplement, 1*, 1–46.

British Association of Counselling Research Committee (1989) Evaluating the effectiveness of counselling. In *A Discussion Document in Counselling, 69*, 27–29.

Brown, G. and Harris, T. (1978) *Social Origins of Depression.* London: Tavistock.

Burnard, P. (1991) *Coping with Stress in the Health Professions.* London: Chapman and Hall.

Byrne, P. (1984) Psychiatric morbidity in a gynaecological clinic: an epidemiological study. *British Journal of Psychiatry, 144*, 28–34.

Chalmers, B. E. and Chalmers, B. M. (1986) Post-partum depression: a revised perspective. *Journal of Psychosomatic Obstetrics and Gynaecology, 5*, 93–105.

Chaplin, J. (1988) *Feminist Counselling in Action.* London: Sage.

Connolly, K. J., Edelmann, R. J. and Cooke, I. (1987) Distress and marital problems associated with infertility. *Journal of Reproductive and Infant Psychology, 5*, 49–57.

Dickson, A. (1982) *A Woman in Your Own Right.* London: Quartet.

Donnai, P., Charles, N. and Harris, R. (1981) Attitudes of patients after genetic termination of pregnancy. *British Medical Journal*, *282*, 621–622.

Dryden, W. and Trower, P. (Eds) (1988) *Developments in Cognitive Psychotherapy*. Newbury Park, C.A.: Sage.

Edelmann, R. J. and Connolly, K. J. (1987) The counselling needs of infertile couples. *Journal of Reproductive and Infant Psychology*, *5(2)*, 63–70.

Egan, G. (1990) *The Skilled Helper*, 4th ed. California: Brooks/Cole.

Eichenbaum, L. and Orbach, S. (1983) *Understanding Women: A Feminist Psychoanalytic Approach*. Harmondsworth: Penguin.

Elliott, S. A. (1989) Psychological strategies in the prevention of postnatal depression. In *Balliere's Clinical Obstetrics and Gynaecology: Psychological Aspects of Obstetrics and Gynaecology*. London: Balliere Tindall.

Elliott, S. A. (1990) Commentary on 'Childbirth as a Reproductive Event'. *Journal of Reproductive and Infant Psychology*, *8*, 147–159.

Fallowfield, L. (1991) Counselling patients with cancer. In H. Davis and L. Fallowfield (Eds) *Counselling and Communication in Health Care*. Chichester: Wiley.

Forrest, G. C. Standish, E. and Baum, J. D. (1982) Support after perinatal death; a study of support and counselling after perinatal bereavement. *British Medical Journal*, *285*, 1475–1479.

Forssman, H. and Thune, I. (1966) 120 children born after application for therapeutic abortion refused. *Acta Psychiatrica Scandinavica*, *42*, 71–83.

Friedman, T. (1989) Women's experiences of general practioner management of miscarriage. *Journal of the Royal College of General Practitioners*, *39*, 456–458

Greene, J. G. and Visser, A. P. (Eds) (1992) Longitudinal studies of the climacteric: special issue. *Maturitas*, *14(2)*, 93–160.

Harris, T. (1967) *I'm OK, You're OK.* London: Pan.

Hawkridge, C. (1987) A survey amongst 800 members of the Endometriosis Society, UK. In *Endometriosis: A Collection of Research Papers*. Coventry: The Endometriosis Society.

Hawton, K., Salkovskis, P. M., Kirk, J. and Clark, D. M. (1989) *Cognitive Behaviour Therapy for Psychiatric Problems: A Practical Guide*. Oxford: Oxford University Press.

Henley, A. and Kohner, N. (1991) *Guidelines For Health Professionals*. London: Stillbirth and Neonatal Death Society.

Hillier, C. A. and Slade, P. (1989) The impact of antenatal classes on knowledge, anxiety and confidence in primiparous women. *Journal of Reproductive and Infant Psychology*, *7*, 3–13.

Hofmeyr, G. J., Nikodem, V. C., Wolman, W-L, Calmers, B. E. and Kramer, T. (1991) Companionship to modify the clinical birth environment: effects on progress and perceptions of labour and breastfeeding. *British Journal of Obstetrics and Gynaecology*, *88*, 756–764.

Holden, J. M., Sagovsky, R. and Cox, J. L. (1989) Counselling in a general practice setting: controlled study of health visitors' intervention in treatment of postnatal depression. *British Medical Journal*, *298*, 223–226.

Hull, M. G. R., Glazener, C. M. A., Kelly, N. J., Conway, D. I., Foster, P. A., Hinton, R. A., Coulson, C., Lambert, P. A., Waall, E. M. and Desai, K. M. (1985) Population study of census, treatment and outcome of infertility. *British Medical Journal*, *291*, 1693.

Hunter, M. S. (1990) *Your Menopause*. London: Pandora.

Hunter, M. S. (1992) The South-East England study of the climacteric and postmenopause. *Maturitas*, *14(2)*, 117–126.

Hunter, M. S. and Coope, J. (1993) *Time of Her Life*. London: BBC Books.

Karmi, G. (1992) *The Ethnic Factfile. The Health and Ethnicity Programme*. North West/North East Thames Regional Health Authorities.

Kirkley-Best, E. and Kellner, K. R. (1982) The forgotten grief: a review of the psychology of stillbirth. *American Journal of Orthopsychiatry*, *52(3)*, 420–429.

Kohner, N. and Henley, A. (1991) *When a Baby Dies*. London: Pandora.

Leventhal, H., Meyer, D. and Nerez, D. (1980) The commonsense representations of illness danger. In S. Rachman (Ed.) *Contributions to Medical Psychology*, Volume 2. New York: Pergamon Press.

Leverton, T. and Elliott, S. A. (1989) Transition to parenthood groups: a preventative intervention for postnatal depression? In E. V. Van Hall and W. Everaerd, (Eds) *The Free Woman: Women's Health in the 1990s*. Carnforth: Parthenon.

Llewelyn, S. (1989) Caring: the costs to nurses and relatives. In A. K. Broome (Ed.) *Health Psychology*. London: Chapman and Hall.

McFarlane, J., Martin, C. L. and Williams, T. M. (1988) Mood Fluctuations: Women Versus Men and Menstrual Versus Other Cycles. *Psychology of Women Quarterly*, *12*, 201–223.

MacLeod Clark, J., Hopper, L. and Jesson, A. (1991) Progression to counselling. *Nursing Times*, *87(8)*, 41–43.

Marteau, T. M. (1989) Psychological costs of screening. *British Medical Journal*, *299*, 527.

Martin, E. (1987) *The Woman in the Body*. Milton Keynes: Open University Press.

Maternity Services (1992) *Health Committee Second Report*. London: HMSO.

Melzack, R. and Wall, P. (1982) *The Challenge of Pain*. Harmondsworth: Penguin.

Nelson-Jones, R. (1988) *The Theory and Practice of Counselling Psychology*. London: Cassell.

Nicholson, P. (1990) Understanding postnatal depression: a mother-centred approach. *Journal of Advanced Nursing, 5*, 689–695.

Nicholson, P. (1989) Counselling women with post-natal depression: implications from recent qualitative research. *Counselling Psychology Quarterly, 2(2)*, 123–132.

Oakley, A. (1979) *From Here to Maternity*. Harmondsworth: Penguin.

Oakley, A. (1988) Is social support good for health of mothers and babies? *Journal of Reproductive and Infant Psychology, 6*, 3–21.

OPCS (1990) *Mortality Statistics: Perinatal and Infant Social and Biological Factors*. England and Wales: OPCS.

Parkes, C. (1978) *Bereavement: Studies of Grief in Adult Life*. Harmondsworth: Penguin.

Payer, L. (1989) *Medicine and Culture*. London: Victor Gollancz.

Pearce, S., Knight, C. and Beard, R. W. (1982) Pelvic pain – a common gynaecological problem. *Journal of Psychosomatic Obstetrics and Gynaecology, 1*, 12.

Pfeffer, N. and Woollett, A. (1983) *The Experience of Infertility*. London: Virago.

Phillips, A. and Rakusen, J. (Eds) (1978) *Our Bodies Ourselves*. Harmondsworth: Penguin.

Pitt, B. (1968) Atypical depression following childbirth. *British Journal of Psychiatry, 114*, 132–143.

Posner, T. and Vessey, M. (1988) *Prevention of Cervical Cancer: The Patient's View*. London: King's Fund Publication.

Ridgeway, V. and Matthews, A. (1982) Psychological preparation for surgery. A comparison of methods. *British Journal of Clinical Psychology, 21*, 271–280.

Riordan, R. J. and Beggs, M. S. (1987) Counsellors and self-help groups. *Journal of Counselling and Development, 65*, 427–429.

Rogers, C. R. (1961) *On Becoming a Person*. Boston: Houghton Mifflin.

Savage, W. (1982) Hysterectomy. London: Hamlyn Paperbacks.

Savage, W., Schwartz, M. and George, J. (1989) *A Survey of Women's Knowledge, Attitudes and Screening in the Tower Hamlets Health District*. Published by authors as a monograph.

Slade, P. (1989) Psychological therapy for premenstrual emotional symptoms. *Behavioural Psychotherapy, 17*, 135–150.

Slade, P., McPherson, S., Hume, A. and Maresh, M. (1990) Expectations and experience of labour. *Journal of Reproductive and Infant Psychology, 8(4)*, 256.

Spielberger, C. D., Gorsuch, R. C. and Lushere, R. E. (1970) *Manual for the Stait-Trait Anxiety Inventory (Self Evaluation Questionnaire).* Palo Alto: Consulting Psychology Press.

Szasz, T. and Hollender, M. (1956) A contribution to the philosophy of medicine: the basic models of the doctor–patient relationship. *Archives of Internal Medicine, 97*, 585–592.

Ussher, J. M. (1989) *The Psychology of the Female Body.* London: Routledge.

Ussher, J. M. (1992) Research and theory related to female reproduction: implications for clinical psychology. *British Journal of Clinical Psychology, 31*, 129–151.

Van Keep, P. A., Wildermeerch, D. and Lehert, P. (1983) Hysterectomy in six European countries. *Maturitas, 5(2)*, 69–77.

Voluntary Licensing Authority (1987) *Second Report For Human In Vitro Fertilization and Embryology.* London: Voluntary Licensing Authority.

Wallace, L. (1984) Psychological preparation for gynaecological surgery. In A. Broome and L. Wallace (Eds) *Psychology and Gynaecological Problems.* London: Tavistock Publications.

Warner, P. and Walker, A. (Eds) (1992) The Menstrual Cycle. Special Issue of *Journal of Reproductive and Infant Psychology,10(2)*, 63–128.

Webb, A. (1989) *Experiences of Hysterectomy.* London: Optima.

Weissman, M. M. and Klerman, G. L. (1981) Sex differences and the epidemiology of depression. In E. Howell and M. Bayes (Eds) *Women and Mental Health.* New York: Basic Books.

Wilson, R. A. (1966) *Feminine Forever.* New York: M. Evans.

Woods, N. F., Olshansky, E. and Draye, M. A. (1991) Infertility: women's experiences. *Health Care for Women International, 12*, 179–190.

Woollett, A. and Dosanjh-Matwala, N. (1990) Asian women's experiences of childbirth in the East End: the support of fathers and female relatives. *Journal of Reproductive and Infant Psychology, 8*, 11–22.

Worsley, A., Walters, W. A .W. and Wood, E. C. (1977) Screening for psychological disturbance amongst gynaecology patients. *Australian and New Zealand Journal of Obstetrics and Gynaecology, 17*, 214.

Index

abortion 22–3, 43, 45
adult–adult model of counselling 52
anger 82–5
antenatal classes 97–9
assertiveness skills 112–3
attention to client 62–6

bad news:
  how to convey 89–92
Beck Depression Scale 130
bereavement 42–8, 100–1
biological factors in reproductive changes 14
biopsy 23–4
biopsychosocial model:
  of counselling 52, 55, 73
  of reproductive changes 3–4, 9–15
brainstorming 58, 110
British Association for Counselling 133
British Psychological Society 134

cancer 42–3
case studies 74–80, 113–122
cervical screening 23–4
childbirth 28–31, 97–9
choices:
  helping clients to make 94–5
client-centred therapy 52–3
cognitive factors in reproductive changes 10
cognitive therapy 55, 57
cognitive-behavioural treatments 99, 131
colposcopy 23
communication 2, 20–1, 49–50, 60, 87, 99,
  102, 129
cone biopsy 23–4
consultation 18–21
contraceptive pill 7
coping strategies 14, 17, 19–20, 96
counselling:
  aims of 50, 130
  definition of 1, 49
  duration of 123–5
  evaluation of 129–132
  goals 57–8, 109–10
  importance of skills 2, 49, 60
  models of 50–2
  process of 52–4
  setting 60–2
  training 69, 85, 103, 132–4
cryocautery 24
cultural differences 4–6, 11, 65

depression 2, 37, 56, 107
diary method 108, 115–16, 130

distress:
  guidelines for dealing with 80–2
doctor–patient relationships 20, 51
donor insemination 32–3

Egan's problem management approach 52,
  54, 59, 108, 124
empathy 16, 53, 66–9
endometriosis 40–1
evaluation of counselling 129–132
expert model of counselling 51

Freud 7

gametic intrafallopian transfer (GIFT) 32
Gate Control Theory of pain 40, 76, 106, 117
genuineness 53
goals 109–10
grief 99–100
  case study of 47, 77–8, 118–20
  stages of 44, 47–8

health promotion 3, 126–7
health workers:
  needs of 132–6
historical changes 6–7
hormones 34–5
hormone replacement therapy (HRT) 7–8, 39
hysterectomy 25–8
  case study of 27–8, 67–8, 78–80, 120–2
hysteria 6

infertility 31–4
information provision 87–97
  guidelines for 88
  medical intervention 92–3
in vitro fertilization (IVF) 32–3

laparoscopy 31, 40–1
laser treatment 24
listening skills 63–5
lithotomy position 23

media image of women 13
menopause:
  attitudes 5, 56
  problems during 37–9
  psychosocial predictors of 38
menstrual taboo 4, 6
menstruation:
  attitudes 4–5

miscarriage 43, 45
mutual participation model of counselling 52, 122

natural childbirth 8
neonatal death 43
    case study of 47, 77–8, 118–120
new perspectives 106–9
non-verbal communication 62–4

oophorectomy 25, 39
open questions 54, 69, 73

pelvic inflammatory disease (PID) 40–1
pelvic pain 40–2
    case study of 18, 75–7, 117–8
perception of symptoms 16–8
perinatal death 46
personality 12, 32, 72
postnatal depression 36–7
post-operative distress 25
pregnancy loss 43–8, 99–103
premenstrual syndrome (tension) 34–5
    case study of 35, 75, 114–6
preparation for surgery 95–7
problem clarification 54–7, 69–72
problem-solving skills 105, 109–112
punch biopsy 23–4
relaxation 93, 108, 112, 125, 140

reproductive cycle problems 34–9
reproductive problems:
    definition of 2
respect 53

self-esteem 13, 39, 56–7, 107
self-help groups 96, 112, 123, 127, 136–9
self-image 5, 12, 42
setting 60–2
sex role stereotypes 13, 107
sexual abuse 2, 13, 55, 74
social expectations 56
social factors in reproductive events 11–12
social support 12, 15, 30, 37, 44, 48
socioeconomic status 11
Spielberger State and Trait Anxiety Scale 130
stillbirth 43, 46
stress management 112–3
summarizing clients' problems 71
supervision 132, 134–5
surgery:
    preparation for 95–7
symptoms:
    perception of 16–8

termination 22–3
training 69, 85, 103, 132–4
transcutaneous nerve stimulation (TENS) 29
twentieth century changes 7–9